EXPERT ENDORSEMENTS

"Here's the big secret laid bare . . . you can't lose weight without building muscle, so follow Jorge's recommendations."

—*Dr. Mehmet Oz, author of* YOU: On a Diet

"Regular physical activity is crucial for weight control and vital for health. But fitting it into our hectic daily routines can seem nearly impossible—until you get some guidance from Jorge Cruise! Jorge is the master of maximum benefit from exercise in minimal time. Read Jorge's latest insights and empowering strategies, and you will discover there *is* time in your life for exercise and its powerful benefits—no heavy lifting required!"

—*David L. Katz, M.D., M.P.H., F.A.C.P.M., F.A.C.P.,*
associate professor adjunct; public health director,
Prevention Research Center Yale University School of Medicine;
medical consultant, ABC News; www.davidkatzmd.com

"Jorge is the embodiment of his own program. This book tells you how to achieve the same results—really great!"

—*Suzanne Somers, #1* New York Times *bestselling author of most recently* Ageless: The Naked Truth About Bioidentical Hormones

"Jorge Cruise's new program will revolutionize how you work out and stay fit. His plan is amazing."

—*Cathleen Black, president, Hearst Magazines, publisher of*
Cosmopolitan, Good Housekeeping, Harper's Bazaar,
O, the Oprah Magazine, *among others*

"Who knew 12 seconds could make such a difference? Jorge Cruise defines how to maximize results in a short amount of time—which is invaluable in this fast-paced world. With traditional strength training, there are reps. With Jorge's program, there are *REPS*! With this technique, you can shape your body faster than you ever thought possible."

—*Kathy Smith, fitness expert and author of* Feed Muscle, Shrink Fat

"I agree with Jorge wholeheartedly. Along with a sound eating plan, strength training is the key to overall health improvement. And, as the saying goes, 'Slow and steady wins the race!' "

—Frederick Hahn, celebrity trainer, author,
and owner of Serious Strength NYC

"Jorge Cruise has done it again! Long at the forefront of teaching people how to live healthy lives, his new book shows you how to exercise effectively, safely, and efficiently. A great guide to a healthier you!"

—John Robbins, author of Healthy at 100 *and the*
internationally acclaimed bestseller Diet for a New America

"I think the 12-Second Sequence™ workout for 20 minutes twice a week in conjunction with the dietary suggestions is the best and most productive way for busy people to get into shape and stay that way. There is no way people could become bored and lose interest in 20 minutes. It reminds me of the commercial quote, 'So easy a caveman could do it.' "

—Dale Eustace, Ph.D., professor of cereal technology,
Kansas State University

"In this chaotic world where dozens of new diet and exercise books seem to pop up every year, it's all too easy to get confused and to give up hope. This book clearly details the 'basics' that should form the foundation to any healthy lifestyle. Read the first few pages and you'll soon discover that you can have the body you've always dreamed of in half the usual time. The 12-Second Sequence™ should be devoured by anyone seeking a common-sense approach to living a great life in a great body."

—Christopher Guerriero, founder of MaximizeYourMetabolism.com
and host of The Energy Factor *health television show*

THE 12-SECOND SEQUENCE™

"The 12-Second Sequence™ works. You'll love the results: boosting your metabolism, increasing your stamina, and easily fitting into your jeans again."

—Lucy Beale, author of The Complete Idiot's Guide to Glycemic Index Weight Loss

"Like me, Jorge Cruise practices what he preaches."

—Jack La Lanne, godfather of fitness and coauthor of Fiscal Fitness: 8 Steps to Wealth & Health from America's Leaders of Fitness and Finance

"Jorge knows what he's talking about. Follow his book—lose the weight."

—Chris Robinson, fitness expert and author of The Core Connection

"Jorge continues to inspire and make losing weight fun and part of your life forever."

—Mariel Hemingway, author of Healthy Living from the Inside Out

THE 12 SECOND SEQUENCE™

SHRINK YOUR WAIST IN 2 WEEKS!

JORGE CRUISE

CROWN PUBLISHERS
NEW YORK

NOTICE

The information given here is designed to help you make informed decisions about your body and health. The suggestions for specific foods, nutritional supplements, and exercises in this program are not intended to replace appropriate or necessary medical care. Before starting any exercise program, always see your physician. If you have specific medical symptoms, consult your physician immediately. If any recommendations given in this program contradict your physician's advice, be sure to consult your doctor before proceeding. Mention of specific products, companies, organizations, or authorities in this book does not imply endorsement by the author or the publisher, nor does mention of specific companies, organizations, or authorities in the book imply that they endorse the book. The author and the publisher disclaim any liability or loss, personal or otherwise, resulting from the procedures in this program. Internet addresses and telephone numbers given in this book were accurate at the time the book went to press.

Product pictures, trademarks, and trademark names are used throughout this book to describe and inform the reader about various proprietary products that are owned by others. The presentation of such pictures and information is intended to benefit the owner of the products and trademarks and is not intended to infringe upon trademark, copyright, or other rights, nor to imply any claim to the mark other than that made by the owner. No endorsement of the information contained in this book has been given by the owners of such products and trademarks and no such endorsement is implied by the inclusion of product pictures or trademarks in this book.

TRADEMARKS

12-Second Sequence	Be in Control
12second.com	Controlled Tension
3-Hour Diet	Jorge Cruise
3-Hour Diet Plate	jorgecruise.com
3hourdiet.com	Time-Based Nutrition
8 Minutes in the Morning	Jorge's Packs

Published in the United States by Crown Publishers, an imprint of the Crown Publishing Group, a division of Random House, Inc., New York.
www.crownpublishing.com

Crown is a trademark and the Crown colophon is a registered trademark of Random House, Inc.

Library of Congress Cataloging-in-Publication Data

Cruise, Jorge.
The 12-second sequence: shrink your waist in 2 weeks / Jorge Cruise. Includes bibliographical references and index.
1. Weight loss. 2. Reducing diets. 3. Exercise. 4. Physical fitness. I. Title. II. Title: Twelve second sequence.
RM222.2.C775 2007
613.2'5—dc22   2007010072

978-0-307-38331-0

Printed in the United States of America

Design by Ruth Lee-Mui

10 9 8 7 6 5 4 3 2 1

First Edition

To my beautiful wife, Heather.
I love you with all my heart.
I am the luckiest man in the world.

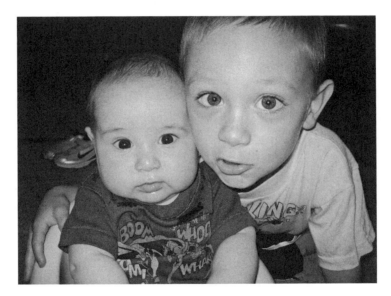

My boys

ACKNOWLEDGMENTS

A very special thank-you to my amazing wife, Heather. She is my most passionate supporter and has helped me become everything I am today. Thank you, sweetheart, for bringing so much inspiration and joy to my life. I love you with all my heart.

To my wonderful sons, Parker and Owen. You both are the light in my eyes. You keep me on my toes and full of wonder as I watch you grow.

To Jared Davis for his tireless work on this book from the very moment of its conception. You have brought your extraordinary fitness, nutritional, and research knowledge to the table and helped me create this project. Thank you so much for helping me to develop and test all the concepts outlined in this book, both in the gym and at home. And then an extra big thank-you for bringing them to life in the photo studio and on video for all our clients. I feel very lucky to have you on our team and to call you a friend.

Thanks to Auriana Albert for her outstanding writing and research abilities, as well as her unwavering commitment to this project. Her creativity and ability to bring the thoughts and concepts to life on paper have been an amazing contribution.

To Gretchen Lees for her endless hours of research and content development. Her amazing writing and research skills helped me substantiate these concepts and provided the facts to support these ideas on paper.

Thanks to Oliver Stephenson and Chance Miles for their exceptional client support. You have helped me manage all our amazing clients who are in this book, stay connected to them, and gather their success stories. Your commitment to our clients and enthusiasm in supporting them is *unsurpassed*. Thank you, guys!

To Chad Wagner for your brain power in data analysis and your ingenuity and skill in creating our extraordinary 12second.com website.

To Trixie Kennedy for keeping us laughing, singing, and paid-up on time. You are a true gem.

To Kathy Thomas, for coordinating all of my projects, tying up all of my loose ends, and for keeping me on track. I am so grateful for your support.

My appreciation also to Steve Hanselman and Cathy Hemming, my literary advisory team at LevelFiveMedia. Steve, thank you for your amazing encouragement, belief, and support for all my projects for the many years I have known you. You were instrumental in helping create a partnership with Random House and for that I thank you as well. To Cathy and Julia Serebrinsky, thank you too for all of your support.

Thanks to Michael J. Dorazio for his spectacular legal support on this project. And of course to my amazing team at Random House who believed in this project from the moment it was laid on the table. Thank you, Heather Jackson, Kristin Kiser, Tina Constable, Jenny Frost, Steve Ross, Christine Aronson, Carrie Thornton, Philip Patrick, Jill Flaxman, Amy Metsch, Linda Kaplan, Andrew Leibowitz, Donna Passannante, Shawn Nicholls, Amanda D'Acierno, Penny Simon, Alison Watts, Milena Alberti, and Sydney Webber.

To Dr. Mehmet Oz for endorsement of this project and friendship. Your extraordinary work is a true force for good and I feel very honored to call you a friend.

My special thanks to Anthony Robbins, Pam Hendrickson, Lisa Sharkey, Dr. David Katz, Jane Friedman, Steve P. Murphy, Ardath Rodale, Bob Wietrak, Edward Ash-Milby, Richard Galanti, Terry Goodman, and Natalie Farage for their outstanding support and friendship throughout the years.

Thank you to Jack Curry and Michele Hatty at *USA WEEKEND* magazine for your extraordinary efforts in helping me get my message out to America every week; I am so grateful for your support and friendship.

And thanks to Cathie Black, Cathy Chermol, Hilary Estey McLoughlin, Tyra Banks, John Redmann, Sheila Bouttier, Katie Couric, Lisa Gregorisch-Dempsey, Meredith Vieira, Amy Rosenblum, Marc Victor, Diane Sawyer, Chris Cuomo, Patty Neger, Monica Escobedo, Wendy Whitworth, Linda Evans, Karen Katz, Emeril Lagasse, Barbara Walters, Bill Geddie, Donald Berman, Dusty Cohen, Cherie Bank, Ivorie Anthony, Jennifer Austin, Kelli Gillespie, and Richard Doutre Jones for allowing me to share my message with the public.

And finally to our newest partners and friends who have provided essential support for this project. Thank you to Jack Hogan, Brian Hogan, Ron Caporale, and Laurie Berger at LifeScript®. To Reid Tracey, Stacey Smith, and Louise Hay at Hay House. To Charles Caswell, Richard Davis, and Paul Goldberg at GoFit™. To Brent Brookes, Jim Zahniser, and Daniel Schwerin at Precor®. To John Wildman, Matt Messinger, and Tia Willows at Bally Total Fitness™. To Bruce Barlean and Jade Beutler at Barlean's Organic Oils. Thanks to Bonnie Block at Fleishman, and Lauren Fritts, Mary Doherty, and Dustin Cohn at Gatorade®.

FROM THE DESK OF JORGE CRUISE

Dear Friend,

The 12-Second Sequence™ is a new way to exercise that will give you maximum results in the least amount of time. It's all about shrinking your waist in two weeks! What's the secret? Well, like my friend Dr. Mehmet Oz emphasizes, it's all about muscle. You see, adding lean muscle tissue to your body is critical to weight loss because it's what drives your metabolism.

"Here's the big secret laid bare. In the long run, you can't lose weight without building muscle, so follow Jorge's recommendations."—Dr. Mehmet Oz, author of *You: On a Diet*

The problem with a lot of other strength-training programs is that they never allow your muscles to achieve maximum fatigue. Too often they focus solely on the quantity of the workout, and not the *quality* of the workout. The 12-Second Sequence™ focuses 100 percent on the *quality* of the exercises. By slowing down each exercise to a 10-second motion and 2-second motionless hold, complete muscle fatigue is achieved and you add sexy, lean, fat-burning muscle to your body faster and more effectively than ever before!

With my new program, you'll be working out **only twice a week for 20 minutes.** You'll notice immediately that this plan is different than anything you've tried before. The very first week, even the very first day, you'll notice your muscles feeling more fatigued than you have after other programs. Your body will become more toned, more firm, and much sexier! Your clothes will fit better and everyone will notice how great you look. Moreover, you'll feel stronger, more fit, and see your waistline shrink within the first two weeks. Visit 12second.com for a free video class with me.

So my challenge to you right now is to commit to this program 100 percent for the first two weeks. Turn to chapter 1 and get motivated to pick up your dumbbells and start the program today. I promise you will see your waist shrink dramatically and you will feel extraordinary. Then, continue the challenge for the remaining six weeks. Bottom line, at the end of the 8-Week Challenge you will look great in a bathing suit! I also want to invite you to join our free $100,000 Challenge for extra motivation. Visit 12second.com for details.

I look forward to seeing you online.

Your coach,

Jorge Cruise

CONTENTS

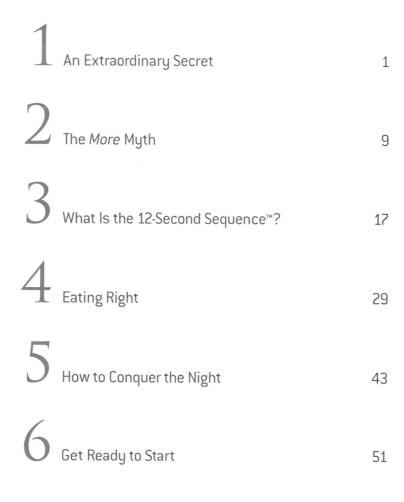

THE 12-SECOND SEQUENCE™

AN EXTRAORDINARY SECRET

1

Life is short, live it well.
—JORGE CRUISE

Something has happened across America, and it's spreading throughout the Western world. People's waistlines are getting bigger and bigger. More than 60 percent of Americans are overweight or obese, and the number keeps growing.

What does this mean for you? Well, if you're overweight—whether you have five or over 30 pounds to lose—you probably aren't living the life you want to lead. Extra weight destroys your self-esteem and truly limits your ability to move freely. Even worse, extra weight around your midsection has been shown to lead to life-threatening health problems like type II diabetes, heart disease, high blood pressure, cancer, and stroke—belly fat is extremely dangerous. I'll discuss why belly fat is so risky in a bit, but for now it's crucial that you realize that getting fit and shrinking your waist are essential to your health.

By the time you finish this chapter, you will understand my extraordinary secret to shrinking your waist in two weeks *and* getting into the best shape of your life. And it will only take two 20-minute workouts each week that you can do at home or the gym. You won't have to spend hours to see results; you'll never waste time on inefficient exercise methods again.

THE KING OF FAT

I know what it's like to feel uncomfortable with your body. I was fat as a kid. My whole family loved to eat huge portions of heavy, rich foods. My mom and grandma believed that a well-fed kid was a well-loved kid—and I would say that I was loved as much as two normal kids combined! I became so chubby that my mom started calling me *el rey,* or "the king" in Spanish. However, my extra fat, my belly fat in particular, was starting to take a huge toll on me, physically and emotionally.

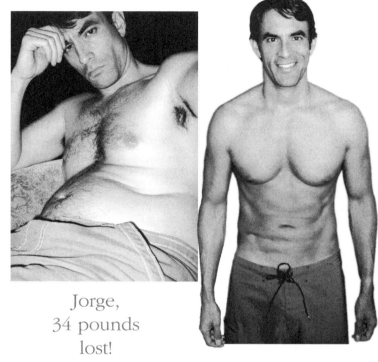

Jorge,
34 pounds
lost!

Exercise was never a priority in my family; my dad worked ten-hour days and considered exercise too difficult and time-consuming. As a result of my poor diet and lack of exercise, I was a mess by the time I was fifteen. I had low energy, daily headaches, and asthma so severe that I wheezed when I tried to run laps in gym class. The other kids in school made fun of me and called me names like "lard-ass" and "fatso." I was never picked for teams. I never played sports, and I couldn't even do one push-up or pull-up. I was so embarrassed by my body that my self-esteem suffered. No one—especially not my family who loved me so much—suspected that my lack of exercise and unhealthy diet were responsible for the challenges I faced.

It took a life-threatening experience to make me realize that my lifestyle choices could kill me. When I was a teenager, my appendix burst and I came within minutes of dying. During the long and difficult recovery period, I began thinking about becoming a healthier person. I realized that I didn't have the tools I needed to start living a healthy lifestyle, but even thinking about it was a big start for me.

Not long after my appendix burst, something happened to my dad that changed both of our lives forever. He was diagnosed with prostate cancer and told that without medical intervention he only had a year to live. Rather than undergo invasive, conventional treatment, my dad enrolled in an alternative health center in San Diego called the Optimum Health Institute to learn how to cleanse, rejuvenate, and heal his body with lifestyle changes. I joined the program with my dad, mostly for emotional support, but I took away life-changing lessons in exercise and nutrition. My dad's cancer went into remission and my headaches and asthma disappeared. We both got healthy and gained energy—as well as a whole new appreciation of life.

My dad wasn't the only member of my family to suffer serious health consequences from his lifestyle choices. My grandparents were both significantly overweight. They didn't think much about their health until my grandmother had a stroke. While she recovered in the hospital, my grandfather got a checkup and learned that his blood pressure was dangerously high. The doctor figured that it was only a matter of time before my grandfather had a stroke, too.

Shaken up, my grandparents decided to learn from my dad's experience at the health center and start leading healthier lives. Unfortunately, it was too late for my grandma; she soon had a second stroke and passed away. However, my grandpa made a lot of beneficial changes even with his grief over losing his wife. He dropped more than fifty pounds and lowered his blood pressure dramatically. He completely turned his health—and his life—around. From that point on, I decided to make my life's mission to become fit and guide others toward longer, healthier, and better lives.

I devoted my time to studying nutrition, exercise science, and psychology. I learned everything I could from my instructors at the University of California, San Diego; Dartmouth College; and the Cooper Institute for Aerobics Research. I also became a certified personal trainer and researched the seemingly endless number of fad diets and exercise programs available. Once I was ready, I set out to create a website that would help online clients get fit. It worked. And soon after, something very big happened—my website and one of my online clients were featured on *The Oprah Winfrey Show*. My life changed after this incredible moment! I received thousands of e-mails from people asking me to help them, too. That inspired me to develop my introductory exercise book series, *8 Minutes in the Morning*. That series of bestselling books was designed for a beginner who just wants a simple plan to get going. Then, at my JorgeCruise.com website, I received more and more e-mails asking me to develop a weight-loss diet that was healthy, safe, and yet still delicious. So I created a book series called *The 3-Hour Diet*. That series got hot fast! For the first time, everyone from college kids to busy moms to celebrities were eating well and seeing results quickly.

This leads me to the book you have in your hands. Yes, as you can imagine, I continued to receive e-mail requests, but this time it was different. People wanted me to create a fitness plan for *maximum results in minimal time—while still keeping it simple.* Specifically, they wanted me to help them shrink their waistlines faster and allow them to achieve their best bodies *ever*. They wanted results that none of my past plans could offer. That pushed me to make an *extraordinary* breakthrough.

A RESEARCH BREAKTHROUGH

Recently, amazing discoveries have been made in exercise physiology. Researchers have discovered that resistance training done just twice a week can specifically help prevent *belly fat*. Yes, resistance training will not only get you toned and fit, but can shrink the most dangerous kind of belly-bulging fat, called *visceral fat*. This kind of deep abdominal fat not only makes us look big and feel uncomfortable, but also can lead to severe health problems.

In fact, a study conducted at East Carolina University found that weight training increased the amount of belly fat burned not only during exercise, but also for 40 minutes after working out! The researchers concluded that not only did weight training burn belly fat, it also prevented fat gain and burned fat throughout the whole body.

In chapter 3, I will share with you all the details about my new program, but for now just know that you no longer have to run a high risk of developing lifestyle diseases like heart disease and diabetes. My goal is to get you to what doctors say is best (and what also looks great in a swimsuit!): a waist circumference under 35 inches for a man or 32.5 inches for a woman. And with the 12-Second Sequence™, I have created a simple and incredibly effective way for you to achieve this.

MY BREAKTHROUGH METHOD: THE 12-SECOND SEQUENCE™

Resistance training is the key to getting you fit because it creates *lean muscle tissue* that burns fat—particularly belly fat. Until now, however, most resistance training programs have been complicated and time-consuming. So that is why my fitness team and I spent two years creating the ultimate fitness plan—*a revolutionary method of resistance training.* And we call that method the 12-Second Sequence™. It's a true breakthrough.

The 12-Second Sequence™ is the most efficient method ever created to develop lean muscle tissue, burn belly fat, and get you looking your best ever. You'll never again waste time in

How Muscle Burns Fat at Rest

If there were a magic wand to help you burn fat and shrink your waist while at rest, it would be lean muscle tissue. You see, lean muscle tissue is metabolically active. What does that mean? Muscle is considered metabolically active because it requires energy to function. In other words, it consumes calories. Fat mass, on the other hand, uses very little energy. In fact, exercise scientist Marla Richmond calls fat a "relatively lazy tissue."

Muscle is the most metabolically active tissue in your body. Muscle sucks up tons of oxygen and other nutrients to feed itself and function optimally. Because it consumes so many calories, muscle is the *number one determinant of your resting metabolic rate.* The more lean muscle tissue you have, the higher your metabolism, and the more calories you burn while doing nothing at all. That is part of the secret to success with the 12-Second Sequence™; keep reading to learn more!

There are many wonderful studies that support the point that your lean muscle mass significantly affects your resting metabolism. One study, conducted by the National Institutes of Health, found that muscle mass is a major contributor to total energy expenditure (calories burned). NIH researchers found that "muscle accounts for 40 to 50 percent of body weight . . . and is therefore, quantitatively, the most important tissue mass on the body."

Lately, some really exciting research has found that increasing your resting metabolism can actually target *belly fat.* Yes, when you increase your metabolism you increase the amount of belly fat you burn while you're doing nothing at all!

An amazing study was recently conducted by the American Heart Association (AHA), which found that strength training could actually prevent belly fat. Researchers found that women who lifted weights two times per week could stop or slow the "middle-aged spread." They studied the effects of increased muscle mass on 164 women aged 24 to 44. After a two-year strength-training program, the women lost almost 4 percent of their total body fat, while participants who did not strength-train lost no body fat. Even more striking was that the women who strength-trained "dramatically reduced the increase in abdominal fat" compared with the group who did not exercise.

Another study, conducted by researchers in Navarra, Spain, found that gains in muscle mass increased resting metabolic rate which, in turn, reduced belly fat. The Spanish researchers studied men with type II diabetes to see if increased muscle mass would have an impact on abdominal fat. At the conclusion of the 16-week training period, the researchers found that the men's average belly fat decreased by about 10 percent! Finally—and this is my favorite study—the University of Alabama at Birmingham subjected fifteen women to a 16-week resistance-training program. At the end of 16 weeks, researchers discovered that the women had "significantly" increased their resting energy expenditure (resting metabolic rate). Moreover, they decreased their abdominal fat by 7.1 percent! Not only did the women in this study trim their waistlines, they also improved their overall body composition and laid the foundation to become more active, healthy people.

the gym doing endless repetitions or spending hours on the treadmill. This workout is so advanced, so to-the-point, that you'll never need another fitness program again.

The 12-Second Sequence™ is made up of two powerful and time-tested workout techniques: slow cadence lifting and static contraction. No other fitness plan has ever combined these two techniques. Slow cadence lifting is a method in which the exercises are slowed down to a 10-second count on the lifting and lowering. With static contraction, the weight or resistance is held at a key point for a predetermined amount of time. I call this unique hybrid technique Controlled Tension™. Although Controlled Tension™ alone is an extraordinary method of training, I still felt that something was missing from the equation.

Recently I became a big fan of circuit training because I discovered that it allowed me to train my entire body in just a few workouts a week and at the same time provided a great cardio workout. In circuit training, you move from exercise to exercise without resting. This allows the heart rate to remain elevated throughout the duration of the workout. And believe me, the cardio benefits are amazing. This final component of the 12-Second Sequence™ makes it the ultimate all-in-one fitness routine.

Bottom line, I believe that the 12-Second Sequence™ is the most efficient, most effective fitness program available. It's the easiest, most realistic program for our culture. America and the rest of the Western world are filled with people just like you and me who want to be fit and healthy, but find it difficult to squeeze an exercise program into our busy lives. Unfortunately our lifestyle has resulted in an overweight, inactive population that suffers from an unprecedented rate of preventable diseases. **It's time to do something about it.** *I want you to live a long, healthy, happy life that's active and fulfilling.* That's why it's so critical that you start this program *today.*

I know that as you embark on your fitness journey with the 12-Second Sequence™, you want to have the best tools and resources available to help sculpt your best body ever. Think of it as you would think of starting to build a home. If you started off with all the wrong materials or the wrong set of plans, you'd have to tear it down and start building all over again. That's why I've done a lot of work for you ahead of time to make sure you have the right "tools" to help you build that beautiful lean muscle and drop belly fat. You'll be able to spot these recommendations when you see my official 12-Second Sequence™ seal of approval that is on the back of this book. This seal means that I trust and believe in these products and companies for their quality, effectiveness, and, most importantly, their ability to help you get to your goal. You will find the official seal on Bally® Total Fitness, where you can get a free 12-Second Sequence™ class when you download the pass from 12second.com; Barlean's® Organic Flaxseed Oils; select GoFit™ equipment; Jorge's Packs™ by LifeScript®; and the Precor® S3.23 functional trainer cable machine and 9.35 treadmill.

So my challenge to you right now is to start the 12-Second Sequence™ 8-Week Challenge. I promise that in the first *two weeks* you will see dramatic results. Not only will your belly shrink, but you'll notice an improvement in your overall fitness level. And at the end of the 8-Week Challenge you will see your best-looking—and best-feeling—body ever!

You'll truly feel the healthiest you've ever felt. You'll feel strong and fit and confident. You'll feel an inner strength such as you've never known before. And you'll look amazing! As you start to create muscle and burn fat, your clothes will become looser and your muscles will become more defined. Everyone will comment on how great you look. And as you burn your belly fat, you will reduce your risk for developing heart disease, diabetes, cancer, and other life-threatening diseases.

Finally, and here's what's most exciting, you'll also increase your *resting* metabolism by up to 20 percent! Yep, you're going to add lean muscle tissue to your body, which will increase the number of calories you burn *at rest*. You're going to train your body to burn hundreds of calories on

How You'll Burn 20 Percent More Calories Every Day

Let's pretend you are an average woman five feet four inches tall, who weighs 160 pounds. This means that you already burn approximately 1,800 calories per day. Ready to boost that? Here's how: On the days that you use the 12-Second Sequence™ (twice per week), you'll burn 200 calories during each workout for a total of 400 calories a week. This boosts your metabolism by 3 percent.

But now the real bonuses start kicking in, and all with *no more* working out. First is the "after-burn," which will burn 200 extra calories after each workout (twice a week) for an additional 400 calories a week. This boosts your metabolism another 3 percent. Yeah!

And then, finally, the best part of all. The 12-Second Sequence™ helps you restore up to five pounds of fat-burning lean muscle tissue. On average, one pound of muscle burns 50 calories per day, so now add an extra 250 calories burned each day or 1,750 more calories burned in a week. This boosts your metabolism further by a whopping 14 percent. I love this!

QUICK OVERVIEW:

      400 calories (from the workout)
      400 calories (from the after-burn)
+ 1,750 calories (from lean muscle tissue)
_____

   2,550 additional calories burned each week! = 20%

Divide that by 7 days in a week and you get *a daily increase of 364 calories* burned or *a 20 percent daily increase in your metabolism!*

its own every week—and that's when you are *not* working out. Imagine burning fat while you sit at your computer or while you sleep! Of all the benefits to my plan, that's my favorite.

Are you ready to change your body? Let's get started.

THE *MORE* MYTH

2

I am working out a lot less than I ever was before, and seeing more results. **When I do the 12-Second Sequence™, in just 20 minutes there are beads of sweat on the muscles I'm working— it is really intense. I am getting the burn, but not the burnout.**

—ROSS COOLING, *12-Second Star, lost 28 pounds*

Y ou've most likely tried everything out there—cardio till you drop, ab machines, traditional weight training, yoga, Pilates, and all the fad workouts. Unfortunately, you most likely discovered that they all require a substantial time commitment before anything happens. This is really frustrating. Most of my clients come to me because they think, "I just don't have the time or energy to get dramatic results, so I'll never be able to get fit."

What people don't realize is that they don't have to spend hours working out every week to get in top shape. In fact, I'm going to introduce you to a vital idea that is going to change the way you think about working out: *more time is not necessarily better.* You've been trapped by the idea that more is better, and this misconception has kept you from achieving your best body ever. *It's crucial that you open your mind to a new way of thinking about exercise, and we'll provide the keys to doing so with the 12-Second Sequence™.*

In this chapter you are going to discover the three biggest myths about getting fit. You need to know these so you never waste your time again. What are they? Many people believe that to achieve the body they want, they need (1) more aerobics *or* (2) more reps *or* (3) more sessions. These techniques can certainly improve your level of fitness, but they're not going to give you that dynamite body you want as effectively as will the 12-Second Sequence™. Learning about these common pitfalls and their weaknesses is the first step toward understanding how this plan will revolutionize your body.

THE MORE-AEROBICS MYTH

Before the 12-Second Sequence™, many of my clients were under the impression that aerobic exercise, like jogging, running, or using an elliptical machine or stair-climber, was the most efficient way to sculpt their ideal bodies. While aerobic exercise is extraordinary for your heart health, it alone will never change the shape of your body as efficiently as resistance training. Consider this: The average person burns about 100 calories for every mile he or she runs. One pound of fat equals 3,500 calories. That means that you have to run 35 miles to burn one pound of fat—just one pound! That is not efficient enough.

Why is cardiovascular exercise not as efficient as strength training when it comes to burning fat? Aerobic exercise lacks a significant "after-burn." I mentioned it in chapter 1, but what exactly is an after-burn? It's the additional calories your body burns *after* you finish a workout. The technical name for after-burn is *excess post-oxygen consumption* (EPOC). During EPOC or the after-burn, your body replenishes its sources of energy, reoxygenates the blood, brings its core temperature back to normal, and returns the heart and breathing rates back to normal. In other words, the after-burn is the effort your body makes to return to homeostasis, which can take several hours. This extra "work" requires your body to burn even more calories than it burned during your workout. Thus the after-burn maximizes your workout by burning calories for hours *after* you stop exercising!

Research has found that resistance training, which again is the heart of the 12-Second Sequence™, alters the body's homeostasis much more dramatically than cardio work. As a result, your body will consume more calories to help it return to normal after lifting weights than after running. This means that you burn more calories for a longer period when you strength-train than when you only do cardio. That is our goal—to rev your metabolism as long as possible to burn fat.

One study at Colorado State University compared the EPOC of a group of test subjects after strength-training exercises and after aerobic exercises. The researchers found that strength training resulted in a significantly higher EPOC, with extra calories still being burned *fourteen and a half hours* after the workout ended. Another study, published in the *International Journal of Sport Nutrition and Exercise Metabolism,* tested the EPOC of women who participated in strength-training exercises. Their average EPOC was 13 percent higher than their pre-exercise oxygen consumption, and this rate stayed elevated for *sixteen hours* after they stopped exercising.

THE MORE-REPS MYTH

If your routine has included resistance training, but you haven't seen the results you wanted, you have probably done *too many* reps and lifted too light a weight. Women, especially, often make the mistake of lifting too-light weights and doing too many reps because they don't want to get big and bulky. This technique is inefficient at getting you to your fitness goals.

For example, a woman who wants to work her triceps may pick up a two-pound dumbbell

Note to Men

Men often believe that the only way to build muscle is to lift very heavy weights. And it's true that lifting heavy weights will cause your muscle tissue to break down. We will discuss this in more detail in chapter 3, as that's not a bad thing; in fact, it's essential to building new muscle. Unfortunately, though, lifting *extremely* heavy weights can be very dangerous and can cause injuries. Even worse, men who are new to working out are often drawn to lifting very heavy weights because it seems like the simplest way to build muscle—and this is where they get into trouble. It can cause injuries from the beginning and soreness beyond what you need to improve your body.

Few people think about the risks involved in lifting very heavy weights. One study published in the *Journal of Sports Medicine* found that weight training can result in fractures, dislocations, herniations, and knee injuries. Why is this type of workout so dangerous? Well, when you lift weights that are too heavy, you aren't able to perform the movements with proper form. Improper form not only increases your risk of injury, but also results in poor muscle development. When you use improper form, you shift the weight burden to smaller muscle groups, and as a result your target muscle doesn't get sufficiently fatigued. I see a lot of men at the gym trying to curl 80-pound dumbbells. The only way they can curl them is to use momentum, straining their backs and taking the weight off the biceps. Working out this way increases your risk of injury and cheats you of an effective workout. The bottom line? You are wasting your time. It looks impressive in the mirror, but it does very little for your body other than hurt it and wear it down.

and do 30 to 40 kickbacks. When she stops, it's not because the exercise was too hard, but because she got bored. She may sweat a bit, get her heart rate up, and feel like she's getting a workout, but it never produces the results she's after. She ends up frustrated and wondering what she's doing wrong. What many women don't realize is that they lack the testosterone hormone necessary to create big muscles. Women produce 30 percent less of this hormone than men, which makes it impossible to bulk up without using dangerous steroids.

Research shows us that when you lift light weights for a lot of reps, you *fail to create the resistance necessary* to build new lean muscle tissue. According to a professor at the West Virginia University School of Medicine, performing 25-rep sets at low or very low intensity will not help you increase your lean muscle tissue. You see, in order to generate muscle tissue, you need to *strain* the muscle so much that you create microscopic tears in the muscle fibers. As your body heals those tears, you generate new lean muscle tissue and become stronger. We'll go into more detail about lean muscle tissue in the next chapter, but for now it's important to understand why lifting light weights will not truly improve your body.

Since lifting light weights doesn't generate enough resistance to build muscle tissue, it's actually closer to a cardio workout than a strength-building workout. What does that mean? No after-burn and no new lean muscle tissue to burn fat! When you lift *light* weights, you burn calories during your workout, but that burn stops when you stop exercising. When you lift light

The Importance of Sleep

Because the 12-Second Sequence™ only requires a 20-minute time commitment, twice a week, you are going to have a lot of extra time on your hands! What should you do with your newfound free time? Get more sleep. Getting enough sleep is more important than you realize. Most people cheat themselves out of a full night's sleep because of stress, home or work responsibilities, or lack of awareness of how important sleep really is. Sleep has a huge impact on your life and health, and it can make a big difference in how you look and feel. When you get eight hours of sleep each night, you give your body a chance to recover and "recharge its batteries." Sleep replenishes growth hormones that are essential to building lean muscle tissue. If you don't get enough sleep, those muscles you worked so hard to tear down don't get a chance to rebuild themselves. As a result, you don't see a change in your body because you're not taking advantage of the body's premium recovery time. Your body actually recuperates best when you get those ideal eight hours of sleep, but, at a minimum, shoot for six hours each night. I know that it might be hard to do, but not sleeping enough is like planting a seed and digging it up every day to see its progress—you're never going to see the fruit or the flower if you don't provide food and rest. This is a lesson that even I have just recently learned—and it has made a great improvement in my life and my body.

weights, therefore, you aren't taking advantage of your body's natural ability to burn calories for hours after you stop working out.

THE MORE-SESSIONS MYTH

And, last but not least, let's talk about how many sessions you do a week—meaning how many workouts you schedule in an average week. Many of my clients believe that to see dramatic results they must do something every day. But when it comes to strength training, all you really need is two sessions a week. That's it! Why? Because if your sessions are intense enough, you will actually need the other five days in the week to let your body rest and recover. Most people don't realize that the only time muscles become stronger and more toned is when they are allowed to rest. If you don't allow your body to rest and recover, you will overtrain and cause more harm than good.

According to the American College of Sports Medicine, "One or more recovery days should be added to each training week." You see, if you don't allow your muscles enough time to recover, they'll never heal and create that strong, lean, shapely look you're after. If you don't rest between training sessions, you undo all your efforts.

Bottom line, it's time to break free from the traditional fitness idea that *more is better*. Methods based on that idea have been wasting your time. And with the 12-Second Sequence™ you will leave failure behind and see your fitness aspirations finally come to life. I challenge you to take this chance to change your life.

So let's get started. Turn the page!

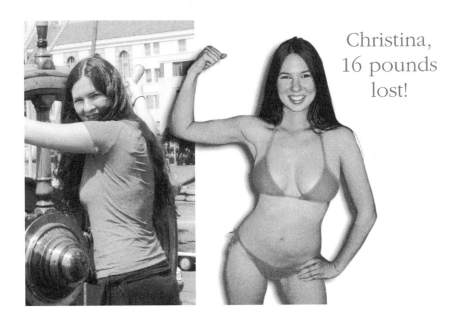

Christina, 16 pounds lost!

12 SECOND STAR

CHRISTINA GECK

Age: 22
Height: 5'5"
Lost: 16 pounds

"Before the 12-Second Sequence™ I had gained weight and I didn't feel comfortable in a swimsuit. My clothes were too tight and I wasn't happy with the way my body felt. "My goal was to look smoking hot in a bikini, and I wasn't sure I could get the beach body I wanted in just 20 minutes, twice a week, but I did. I feel like a Victoria's Secret model now—I'm ready for the runway or at least the beach!

"I love the workouts because they were highly effective and fit very well into my schedule. I definitely notice a difference in the way my body looks and the way I feel—and the best thing is, my body changed and I saw great improvements in such a short time.

"My clothes actually fit me now rather than being too tight, and I feel great when I look in the mirror. I feel hot again!"

CHRISTINA'S SECRETS TO SUCCESS

· Have a friend to keep you on track.
· Plan what you're going to eat every day.
· Don't give up.

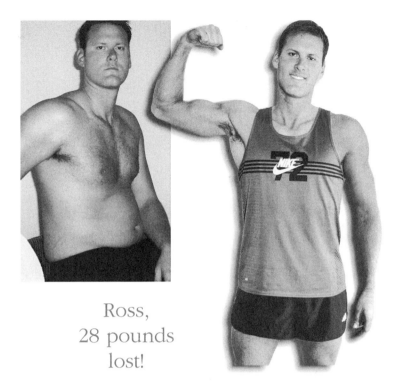

Ross,
28 pounds
lost!

"Before the 12-Second Sequence™, not a day went by that I didn't think about my weight and how unhappy I was with my body. I tried numerous diet and exercise programs, including Atkins, Body-*for*-LIFE, and Weight Watchers, but nothing worked.

"The 12-Second Sequence™ has inspired a complete lifestyle change for me. I feel incredible and have a lot more energy. Best of all are the compliments that I get from friends, family, and even strangers. Before the 12-Second Sequence™, my lifestyle was out of balance and unhealthy. I was continuously overeating, over-exercising, and undersleeping. I feel much more alive and able to enjoy life now!"

ROSS'S SECRETS TO SUCCESS

· Plan and schedule a specific time for your two weekly workouts.
· Each night, cook your meals and prepare your snacks for the next day and store them in to-go containers.
· Visualize a time when you were happy with your body—or just happy with your life. Remember the confidence and attention that came with it, and make that a motivator as you progress through the 12-Second Sequence™.

WHAT IS THE 12-SECOND SEQUENCE™?

3

The very first week, I felt stronger, more fit, and more alive. Best of all, I noticed that I was getting more attention and admiring looks from other people!

—ANNABELLE ESPIRITU, *12-Second Star, lost 13 pounds*

Well, the time has come to reveal my breakthrough method to rev your metabolism by 20 percent every day, shrink your waist, and get your best-looking body ever—all in just two simple 20-minute workouts that you can do at home or at the gym. Are you ready? Let's get started!

HOW IT WORKS

The secret to what makes the 12-Second Sequence™ so efficient and how it will produce such dramatic visible results is my trademarked technique, *Controlled Tension*™, which I mentioned in chapter 1. No other fitness program uses Controlled Tension™. It's the magic that makes this plan so revolutionary. You see, in order to generate *new* fat-burning lean muscle tissue in the least amount of time, you must fully engage *all three types* of skeletal muscle fibers during the same workout. Skeletal muscles are simply the muscles on your body that you can see. Yes, they are the ones we want to tone and work out. The problem is that most resistance training methods don't allow this to happen ever, let alone in just 20 minutes.

With Controlled Tension,™ you will recruit all three muscle fiber types and discover **the real secret to effectively creating lean muscle tissue in such a short amount of time**—*full muscle saturation.* What exactly is full muscle saturation? It simply means fatiguing all three types of skeletal muscle fibers. When you perform an exercise, your brain sends signals to the muscle fibers that are needed to help out. This is called *muscle fiber recruitment.* When all of them are there to help, you are getting the most powerful, amazing workout— and you are creating your fat-burning lean muscle faster than you ever thought possible.

2 seconds

10 seconds

Controlled Tension™ is the key to the 12-Second Sequence™.

Most other resistance training methods don't engage all three fiber types, which makes them less effective in transforming your muscle tissue. But Controlled Tension™ does. It's truly a revolution- ary, hybrid resistance-training method that will *guarantee* full muscle saturation. By combining slow cadence lifting and static contraction, we have developed the ultimate hybrid technique. For the first time ever, these two uniquely efficient techniques are combined into one simple, quick, effective exercise method. Let's take a quick look at what these techniques are, and why they're so darn effective.

SLOW CADENCE LIFTING

In the early 1980s, the University of Florida conducted a clinical trial to see if strength training could help older women with osteoporosis regain lost bone mass. In the study they realized that traditional training with explosive movements could damage weakened joints and bones and possibly do more harm than good. So they decided to slow the movements down to a 10-second "cadence" lift and a 10-second "cadence" return to the starting position. The results were outstanding. Not only was this technique kinder on the joints, but they also found that their test subjects increased lean muscle tissue more quickly than with conventional weight training.

In 2003 another series of studies once again revealed the power of slow cadence lifting. First some prominent physicians at Colorado State University acknowledged the incredible benefits of slow cadence lifting, praising its efficiency and its safety as a workout method. Then the Harvard Medical School endorsed another program that implemented the slow cadence movement. They found that this way of working out was the first to truly show results in such a short amount of time.

Several other research studies support the slow cadence lifting technique. One study, published in the *Journal of Sports Medicine and Physical Fitness,* compared the effects of conventional strength training and slow cadence lifting on muscle growth. They found that the slow-lifting technique increased muscle strength in men and women by about 50 percent more than conventional training.

Another study, published in the *Journal of Exercise Physiology,* evaluated how much impact momentum had on the effectiveness of a strength-training exercise. That study found that unless constant tension is applied to the muscle, muscle force (how many fibers are recruited) decreases as the momentum increases. It's necessary, the study concluded, to maintain deliberate and controlled tension on the muscle to recruit the maximum number of fibers.

Bottom line, when you slow down your workout you minimize the momentum that would normally help you lift weights in conventional strength training. By eliminating the momentum, you target and engage each and every muscle fiber until they all help you perform an exercise. You achieve full muscle saturation faster than you ever thought possible. And the result? You create, tone, and define your fat-burning lean muscle in record time.

STATIC CONTRACTION

The other key component of Controlled Tension™ is what's known as *static contraction.* I first learned about static contraction from my good friend and mentor Tony Robbins. He wrote the foreword to my first book, *8 Minutes in the Morning,* as well as to a book called *Max Contraction Training: The Scientifically Proven Program for Building Muscle Mass in Minimum Time.* According to Tony, "In such a short period of time, in comparison to conventional workouts, [with static contraction training] you can increase your quality of life, look good, feel good . . . and even reduce your stress levels and overall amount of body fat."

So what exactly is static contraction? Well, it actually has the same goal as slow cadence lifting—to achieve full muscle saturation. But rather than using a slow movement, static contraction is based on a motionless hold that stimulates all three muscle fibers, which results in full muscle saturation. You see, muscles only do two movements—contract or extend. According to the static contraction method, when you hold a heavy weight in a muscle's fully contracted state for a given duration (usually one to six seconds), you recruit the absolute maximum number of muscle fibers. The bottom line is that you do very hard work for a short period and see significantly greater muscle growth than with conventional training.

Like slow cadence lifting, the effectiveness of static contraction is supported by numerous research studies. Some of the original research was done by a doctor in Germany who discovered that his test subjects increased their strength by up to 5 percent each week. Another study, done by the authors of a book called *Static Contraction Training,* produced phenomenal results. They subjected volunteers who had been weight-training for over two years to a static-contraction training program for ten weeks. They found that the participants' average strength increased by an amazing 51 percent! Moreover, those who saw the highest gains in strength and muscle mass were those who worked out the least! They averaged just two workouts per week. This study proved that not only is it beneficial to work out at a higher intensity less frequently, but also that maximum muscle contraction stimulates more muscle fibers than conventional training. The result? Great gains in strength and lean muscle mass.

Now, you may have noticed that the last study I mentioned involved people who had been strength-training for a while already. They were doing what I would call traditional static contraction, which isn't always very practical because it requires a gym for every workout, a training partner, and long-term time commitment. And the truth is, unless you are a professional athlete, lifting the kind of weight they were working with can be very dangerous. And yet, static contraction is such a powerful technique, because it promotes full muscle saturation, that we had to figure out a way to modify it for people like you and me. Now, with my Controlled Tension™ method, nearly everyone can benefit from the powerful and effective techniques of slow cadence lifting and static contraction.

CIRCUIT TRAINING

Circuit training is the bonus component of the 12-Second Sequence™. You know that Controlled Tension™ combines slow cadence lifting with static contraction to recruit the maximum number of muscle fibers and build the most muscle. To maximize your workout even further, I added a third component to the 12-Second Sequence™ called *circuit training,* in which a series of exercises are arranged consecutively, and the person moves from exercise to exercise without resting between sets. Circuit training is a crucial component of the 12-Second Sequence™ because it ensures that you work your whole body in those two 20-minute weekly sessions. Moreover, it adds a vital cardiovascular dimension to your routine that gets your heart rate up and helps you burn more calories.

A lot of evidence supports the value of adding circuit training to your fitness regimen. One study, published in *The Physician and Sports Medicine,* found that circuit training increased muscular strength up to 32 percent and decreased body fat up to almost 3 percent among its volunteers. Another study, published in the *Scandinavian Journal of Medicine and Science in Sports,* subjected twelve men to ten weeks of circuit weight training. They found that circuit weight training improved muscular strength and increased lean muscle mass among all of the participants more significantly than conventional weight training.

Furthermore, a study published in the *Journal of Strength and Conditioning Research* found that strength training in a circuit improved cardiovascular fitness. Researchers tested volunteers for basic strength and cardiovascular fitness and subjected them to strength-training exercises within a circuit. They concluded that the stress inflicted on the body by weight training within a circuit was "substantial enough to stimulate a cardiovascular training response." This means that working your muscles in a circuit does more than increase your strength and muscle mass—it also improves the health of your heart and lungs.

And finally, in the study that I love the most, university researchers in Korea found that aerobic training combined with resistance training—circuit training—decreased fat, particularly *belly fat,* better than did aerobic training alone. The researchers divided a group of 30 obese women, aged 40 to 45, into three groups. One group did only cardiovascular exercise, another group did resistance training combined with cardio, and the third group did no exercise. At the end of 24 weeks, the researchers found that the control group increased their body fat percentage. The aerobic-only group lost body fat but did not increase their lean body mass. The combined-exercise group significantly increased their lean body mass and decreased their body fat percentage. **In fact, the combined-exercise group lost two and a half times as much belly fat as the aerobic-only group!** The researchers concluded that circuit training can reduce belly fat more effectively than aerobic activity alone.

Morning Cardio

One way to accelerate your results on the 12-Second Sequence™ is to add cardio to your routine. You might be thinking, But, Jorge, I thought cardio was built into the 12-Second Sequence™ program! You're right, cardio is built into the program with the circuit-training element. However, adding separate bonus cardio, especially first thing in the morning on an empty stomach, will really help you burn off those unwanted pounds fast. I consider it *bonus* cardio because you don't have to do it to see results. It will, however, speed up your results and give you your best body even faster. It's kind of like extra credit—morning cardio on an empty stomach will get you to a grade A+ body!

All you have to do is take a brisk walk for 20 minutes each morning on an empty stomach. The bonus cardio plan is going to help you burn an additional 150 to 200 calories a day. Let's say you walk before breakfast six times a week. That's up to *1,200 more calories a week* you could be burning. That means you'll lose those unwanted pounds and reveal your shapely new body *even faster*.

Several research studies support the concept that morning cardio on an empty stomach is incredibly effective. One study done at Kansas State University compared the number of calories people burned when they exercised before eating and an hour after eating. They found that the actual amount of calories burned did not differ that much, but that those who exercised before eating actually burned "*significantly more fat*" than those who waited until after they ate. The key is to get your walk in before you eat.

Another study conducted at the University of California at Berkeley confirmed this by finding that fat loss increased *only* when the study participants "exercised in a fasted state." Your body fasts at night when you are sleeping and your metabolism naturally slows down because you just don't need as much energy when you are asleep. So when you get your energizing walk first thing in the morning, you rev your metabolism from the very start of your day.

Bottom line: A brisk walk first thing in the morning will burn more fat and get you to your goal even faster than the strength-training exercises alone.

HOW TO DO THE 12-SECOND SEQUENCE™

Now let me give you a simple overview of how the program works. Chapter 6 will give you the full details you need to get started, but right now I want to familiarize you with what the program is and briefly how to do it.

Each workout is divided into three circuits, with four exercises in each circuit. You will do four reps of each exercise. Each exercise begins with the weight or resistance being lifted or lowered slowly and controlled to a count of 10 seconds (the slow-lifting component) until you reach what I call the *maximum tension point* (MTP). The maximum tension point is the key position in the exercise where gravity and the nature of the exercise itself have the most beneficial effect on the muscle. At this strategic point, the weight or resistance is concentrated and squeezed to a strict count of two whole seconds (the static contraction component). *This is where the 12-Second Sequence™ got its name; the 10 seconds of controlled movement plus a 2-second static hold equals 12 seconds of the most intensive weight training you've ever experienced.* Then, to a count of ten, you slowly return to the starting position and, without pausing, begin the next rep. When you finish one set, move smoothly to the next exercise without resting between sets.

Each circuit in the 12-Second Sequence™ is carefully constructed to work your whole body in two 20-minute workouts per week. On Day 1, you'll work your primary muscles—legs, back, chest, and abs. On Day 2, you'll work your secondary muscles—shoulders, biceps, triceps, and abs. You'll notice that we work abs on both days, and there's a very specific reason why. Abs are a more resilient muscle group than others, which means that it takes less time than your biceps or your quadriceps for your abs to heal. We take advantage of the abs' natural ability to heal quickly to build muscle as efficiently as possible.

WORKOUT SCHEDULE

M	T	W	Th	F	S	Sun
Primary muscles: legs, back, chest, and abs			**Secondary muscles:** shoulders, biceps, triceps, and abs			

There are a couple of ways to track your workouts. There are special sheets in the resources where you can log your workouts. These logs will be useful in helping to make sure you do your workouts and in reminding you of your commitment. See handwritten samples on the following pages. When you look back on all the workouts you've completed, you'll feel so proud, and you'll be motivated to continue to the end. In addition, there's a special grid that you can download from 12second.com that will help you track both your workouts and your eating. It includes helpful hints on ideal fats, proteins, and carbs, as well as calorie guides. Also, you can pick up a copy of the *12-Second Sequence™ Journal,* which includes your Workout Logs, Eating Planner, and space for journaling, as well as motivational quotes and visualizations. Whichever method of tracking your progress you choose, pick one that you'll stick with. That way, you're sure to be successful!

That's it! That's the 12-Second Sequence™. Although it might sound simple, it is intense. These exercises will stress your muscles beyond what you may have done before—but they will do so safely and more effectively than any other workout. When you do the 12-Second Sequence™, you'll notice immediately that this workout is different from any you've tried before. The very first week, even the very first day, you'll notice your muscles feeling more fatigued than they have after other exercise programs. Your body will become more toned and firm, and much more shapely. Your clothes will fit better and everyone will notice how much better you look. Moreover, you'll soon feel stronger, more fit, and in better health than ever before.

It's critical that you commit *right now* to my 8-Week Challenge and start creating the body you've always wanted. Remember, in just the first two weeks you will see your waist shrink dramatically! Chapter 6 will share more details with you. I want you to commit yourself to this challenge and watch your ideal body emerge in less time than you thought possible. Remember, when you commit to the 12-Second Sequence™, you're going to build lean muscle to burn the maximum number of calories at rest.

Let's get started!

Primary Workout			
DATE___1/7___ DAY___1___ OF 56	Start>time___7:00___ Finish>time___7:20___ TOTAL TIME___20 minutes___		

Select weights so that by the end of the 4th rep of each exercise you feel an intensity level of 8.

	Muscle Group	Exercise	Weight Used	Intensity Level
CIRCUIT 1	LEGS	beg. squat	N/A	6
	BACK	pullover on Swiss ball	5	8
	CHEST	incline on Swiss ball	10	8
	ABS	curl-up crunch	N/A	8

At this point you should be about 6 minutes into your workout.

	Muscle Group	Exercise	Weight Used	Intensity Level
CIRCUIT 2	LEGS	Swiss ball squat	N/A	7
	BACK	bent-over rows	10	8
	CHEST	push-up on knees	N/A	8
	ABS	chair crunch	N/A	8

At this point you should be about 14 minutes into your workout, including 2 minutes of transition time.

	Muscle Group	Exercise	Weight Used	Intensity Level
CIRCUIT 3	LEGS	plié squat	5	6
	BACK	hyperextension	N/A	8
	CHEST	flat dumb. fly	5	8
	ABS	broomstick twist	N/A	8

At this point in your workout you should be at 20 minutes. Congratulations! YOU DID IT!

BONUS CARDIO 26-MINUTE MORNING POWER WALK ●

After my workout I feel___energized___

(e.g., confident, strong)

Secondary Workout

DATE ___1/10___ DAY ___4___ OF 56

Start>time ___7:30___ Finish>time ___7:50___

TOTAL TIME ___20 minutes___

Select weights so that by the end of the 4th rep of each exercise you feel an intensity level of 8.

CIRCUIT 1

Muscle Group	Exercise	Weight Used	Intensity Level
SHOULDERS	standing shoulder press	10	8
BICEPS	standing curl	10	8
TRICEPS	chair dip	N/A	8
ABS	toe reach	N/A	7

At this point you should be about 6 minutes into your workout.

CIRCUIT 2

Muscle Group	Exercise	Weight Used	Intensity Level
SHOULDERS	standing lat. raise	10	8
BICEPS	side curl on Swiss ball	10	8
TRICEPS	dumb. skull crusher	5	7
ABS	Swiss ball crunch	N/A	8

At this point you should be about 14 minutes into your workout, including 2 minutes of transition time.

CIRCUIT 3

Muscle Group	Exercise	Weight Used	Intensity Level
SHOULDERS	seated rear delt raise	5	7
BICEPS	preacher curl on ball	10	8
TRICEPS	standing tri. kickback	10	8
ABS	lying obl. twist	N/A	8

At this point in your workout you should be at 20 minutes. Congratulations! YOU DID IT!

BONUS CARDIO 26-MINUTE MORNING POWER WALK ●

After my workout I feel ___motivated___

(e.g., confident, strong)

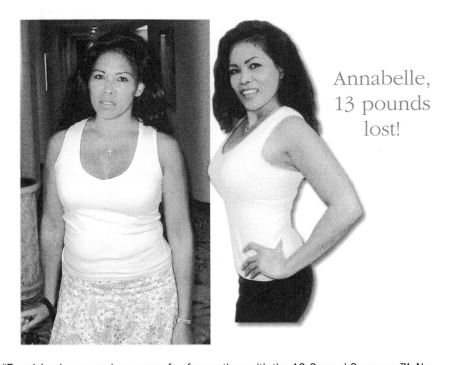

Annabelle, 13 pounds lost!

"Exercising has never been more fun for me than with the 12-Second Sequence™. No more trying to figure out what machines to use and what exercises to do, since all I have to do is follow the circuits. I have invested minimal time and seen fantastic results in such a short period of time—I am even able to get back into my skinny jeans!

"Other people are also noticing the amazing changes in my body. I am forty-eight years old and I want my modeling body back—it's almost there! I have noticed my backside slimming down; my legs are getting back those great curves they used to have, and my arms are getting more defined and sexy. And let's not forget the stomach area—it is tightening and visibly flatter. I am hooked on the 12-Second Sequence™ for life."

ANNABELLE'S SECRETS TO SUCCESS

· Eat a lot of veggies.
· Have a healthy breakfast every day (I like to have a salad!).
· Believe that you're worth the effort.

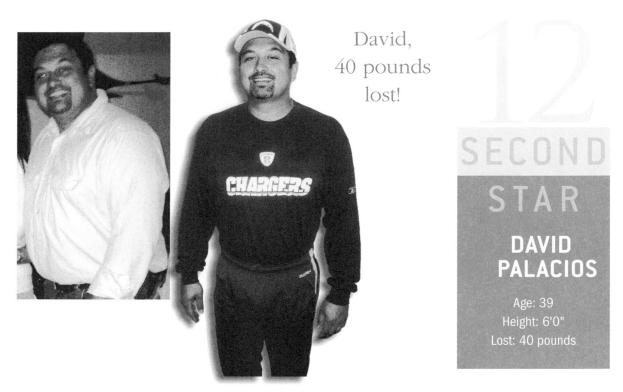

David,
40 pounds
lost!

"When I first started the 12-Second Sequence™, I was very sluggish and my blood pressure was always high. I was constantly being asked, 'Why are you breathing so hard?' I couldn't keep up with my two-year-old son who always wanted to play. I took the challenge for him and my baby daughter—I wanted to feel good for me and my whole family.

"I have lost 40 pounds in just eight weeks. I don't feel sluggish anymore—in fact, I feel light on my feet! I don't get winded after playing with my son for just five minutes. I love the compliments and I feel much more confident and attractive. Even more, I developed great muscle definition and lost so much fat from my stomach, I had to buy new pants!"

DAVID'S SECRETS TO SUCCESS

· Do your exercises with intensity.
· Eat lots of vegetables and salads first, and then your meat and potatoes.
· Love yourself enough to make a change.

EATING RIGHT 4

Using Jorge's eating plan helped me take control of my eating and lose over 150 pounds! It allowed me to become an active participant in my life, instead of just a spectator. **I am now feeling ab muscles where I haven't had any for more than fifteen years!**

—MELODIE RICHARDSON, *12-Second Star, lost 161 pounds*
(combined with the 3-Hour Diet™)

Many of my clients think that if they are exercising, they don't have to care about what they eat. But what you eat *does* matter. It's critical to your success. Think about baking a cake. What do you need to make a delicious cake on the first try? Two main things: a proven recipe and the actual ingredients, like eggs and flour. Right? Well, when it comes to creating lean muscle tissue the same is true. Imagine the 12-Second Sequence™ as the proven recipe, and think of your diet as the ingredients that will literally construct your new body.

Knowing how to eat right will ensure that you whittle your waist and achieve your best body ever. In this chapter I've put together a plan that's simple to follow. It's a plan based on my 3-Hour Diet™ method of eating every three hours. On this new plan, however, you'll consume additional protein to make sure that you're able to build new muscle tissue. This means that your diet will be made up of 40 percent protein, 40 percent carbs, and 20 percent fat. You can set aside all mathematical calculations. In this book I have done all the work for you. Follow this eating plan and you are guaranteed to see results from every one of your 12-Second Sequence™ workouts. It will ensure that you look your absolute best in the least amount of time.

SAMPLE DAY

Breakfast 7 a.m.	Snack 10 a.m.	Lunch 1 p.m.	Snack 4 p.m.	Dinner 7 p.m.	Bedtime Snack 10 p.m.
3 whole eggs, scrambled, two 1-ounce turkey slices (if you weigh over 150 pounds), ⅛ avocado, 1 whole wheat tortilla, and 1 apple	1 whey protein shake	3 to 5 ounces lean chicken, ½ cup brown rice, and a green salad with 1 teaspoon flaxseed oil	1 whey protein shake	3 to 5 ounces grilled steak, a double serving of steamed broccoli, plus a green salad with 1 teaspoon flaxseed oil	1 whey protein shake

See Protein section for recommended protein amounts based on your weight.

THE FIRST SECRET: TIMING

With my eating plan, you will eat breakfast within one hour of rising, and three hours later you'll eat your first snack. Three hours after that, you'll eat lunch. Three hours after lunch, you'll eat your afternoon snack, followed by dinner—you guessed it—three hours later. Before you go to bed, you'll eat your last snack. Each meal ranges from approximately 400 calories to 600 calories, depending on your weight, and each snack is approximately 100 calories. But you will not have to count calories. Again, I have done the work for you.

Why is eating every three hours so powerful in helping you restore lean muscle tissue? Well, I wrote a whole book series on that concept, which I mentioned in chapter 1, called the

3-Hour Diet™. In a nutshell, it will help you do three *vital* things: reduce your cortisol hormone levels, which contribute to belly bulge; keep your metabolism elevated so you stay energized and continue to burn fat; and help control your appetite so you don't overeat and bury your muscles in fat. This is such a vital secret, I promise it will dramatically increase the success you see. For more details, feel free to visit our 3HourDiet.com website.

THE SECOND SECRET: MUSCLE-MAKING INGREDIENTS

So what are you eating every three hours? No food group has been removed. I don't believe in deprivation, because it just leads to cravings and binges. You will eat protein, of course, but you will also eat carbohydrates and fat. *The key is to eat these foods in the right amounts, so that you hit a 40/40/20 "end of day" ratio.*

Again, that means that 40 percent of your calories should come from protein, 40 percent from carbs, and 20 percent from fat. These are the ideal quantities of macronutrients to ensure that you get your best body ever in the shortest amount of time. If you have specific health concerns or nutritional requirements, be sure to consult your doctor before beginning this program.

Let me briefly share with you what these nutrients are, and why they're so crucial to your success on this program.

Protein

The word *protein* derives from the Greek word *prota,* which means, "of primary importance." Protein is the principal building block for all your body's tissues, especially your lean muscle tissues. Protein is made up of chains of molecules called amino acids. What happens if we don't get enough of these amino acids? Our cells seek nutrients from our lean muscle tissue instead of our food, and cannibalize it to repair other tissues in the body. That must be avoided, and getting enough protein each day is the secret.

For the 12-Second Sequence™ eating plan, you want to choose low-fat, high-quality protein as often as you can. My top choices are white meat chicken and turkey (breast, not thigh), lean beef, pork tenderloin, all kinds of cold-water fish, and eggs. (Compared to high-fat proteins like beef, fish and eggs are relatively low in fat. Fish is high in good fat, and eggs do have some saturated fat. However, the pros of their high-quality protein outweigh the cons of their fat.) You can also include low-fat dairy products like 1-percent or skim milk, cottage cheese, and yogurt. Choosing lean sources of protein will help keep your calories down so you can reach your best body in minimal time. Portion size is important also. **If you weigh under 150 pounds, eat 3 ounces of protein at every meal; if you weigh more than 150 pounds, eat 5 ounces of protein.**

In addition to consuming protein with your three main meals, I want you to consume snacks between your meals in the form of **whey protein** shakes. Whey is a high-quality, rich source of protein that's packed with nutrients and essential amino acids. *This is why whey protein has the highest biological value (BV) of all protein sources.* That means that your body will absorb it more readily than other sources of protein. Since your body can digest whey so easily, your muscles can use it right away to repair and create new tissue. As a result, you'll have the greatest nutritional advantage to create the lean and defined body you're after.

There's one more thing you need to know about whey protein. It comes in three different forms: concentrate, isolate, and hydrolysate. Whey protein concentrates contain about 29 percent to 89 percent pure protein and have some fat and carbohydrates. Whey protein isolates contain about 90 percent to 95 percent pure protein and have been processed to remove the lactose and fat. Whey protein hydrolysates are isolates that have been predigested, which means that the proteins have been broken down into smaller pieces so the body can absorb them more easily.

PROTEIN SOURCE	BV
Whey protein	100–159
Whole egg	88–100
Cow's milk	91
Egg white	88
Casein	80
Soy protein	74
Beef protein	80
Wheat gluten	54

SOURCES
Protein Quality Evaluation, Report of the Joint FAO/WHO Consultation and *Reference Manual for U.S. Whey Products,* 2nd edition, U.S. Dairy Export Council.

In addition to helping you build lean muscle, whey protein has tons of health benefits. It can help reduce the risk of developing preventable illnesses, like cardiovascular disease. It has been found to help prevent or reduce high blood pressure and cholesterol, which are among the leading causes of heart disease and stroke. Whey protein has also been associated with lower rates of certain cancers. High levels of cysteine found in whey protein have been correlated with lower risk of developing breast and prostate cancers. Whey protein is also high in immunoglobulins, alpha-lactalbumin, and beta-lactalbumin, all of which boost your immune system. Just one more reason to make sure you drink your whey protein shakes!

Now, you might be wondering what kind of whey protein to look for. I've looked for years for one that tastes great and is easy to use—and it hasn't been easy to find one with the right combination. That's why I'm so excited to tell you about a great new whey protein I've helped create. I've teamed up with a cutting-edge company called LifeScript® to take all the guesswork out of it. We've created Jorge's Packs™—whey protein powder packets that are available exclusively online at jorgepacks.com and delivered right to your door. It tastes great and comes in three different flavors: chocolate, vanilla, and strawberry. We've also developed customized single-serving vitamin packets that contain everything else you'll need for one day—including a daily multivitamin and any other essential supplements that may be right for your personal nutritional needs.

Carbohydrate

Carbs are very important on this eating plan, too. The trick is to know which carbs to eat and when. For your breakfast and lunch, your goal is to focus on whole carbs and minimize refined, or simple, carbs. Whole carbs are your best friend because they contain large amounts of *fiber*. Fiber is good for you because it helps you feel full longer, so you don't eat as much throughout the day. Also, since you can't digest it, fiber sweeps through your digestive system ("nature's broom") and keeps things moving smoothly. Fiber keeps you regular, in good digestive health, and helps reduce the risk of developing colon cancer.

You can find good carbs in foods like fruits, vegetables, and whole grains. Good sources of whole grains include whole grain bread, brown rice, and products made with whole wheat flour. At breakfast and lunch, aim to have ½ cup of starchy carbs or 1 slice of bread. Fruits and veggies (especially green leafy ones) are excellent sources of carbohydrates that are rich in vitamins and minerals. At least half your plate (about 2 cups) at breakfast and lunch needs to be filled with these kind of non-starchy carbs.

My last note on carbs is that on this plan you'll *stop eating starchy carbs after your afternoon snack*. For breakfast and lunch, you will eat starchy ones like toast, brown rice, potatoes, or pasta. However, eat only nonstarchy vegetables with your dinner, like salad greens, spinach, green beans, or zucchini. No potatoes! This is important because as you become less active in the evening, you will not need the high energy that carbs provide. They'd most likely be stored as fat, and we want to avoid that. Have a double serving of broccoli for dinner or add a big green salad. Or try my recipe for pureed cauliflower on page 200. You'll never miss the carbs.

Fat

A lot of people think *fat* is a scary word. But not so. Fat can be your friend. You see, certain essential fats are crucial to helping the body create lean muscle tissue. Essential fatty acids (EFAs) called *omega fats* truly aid the body in creating tissues—primarily muscle tissue, but also hair, skin, and nails. They even help keep your joints healthy. If you focus on eating pri-

Avoid the Fat Trap

To avoid unhealthy fats, you need to understand what types of food they hide in. Here are some examples for two specific types of bad fats.

Saturated fats. These are found in high amounts in animal products such as beef, milk, cheese, lunch meat, butter, and bacon. You can avoid these fats—and continue to eat animal products—if you:

· Choose lower-fat options such as white meat chicken and turkey without the skin, and reduced-fat dairy products. Even with red meat, look for the lowest-fat options (ground sirloin or round, sirloin steaks, reduced-fat lunch meat, reduced-fat bacon and ham). I also recommend that you try soy versions of traditional meat—they taste great and are much lower in fat.
· Watch your portion size. Hold yourself to a 3- to 5-ounce serving of meat per meal (3 ounces if you weigh under 150 pounds; 5 ounces if you weigh over 150 pounds), roughly the size of one or two decks of cards.

Trans fats. Also called partially hydrogenated fats, trans fats are the worst kinds of fat you can eat. Trans fats clog your arteries, lower your good cholesterol, and raise your bad cholesterol. Try to avoid these as much as possible. These fats can be found in just about all processed foods. Common trans-fat culprits include biscuits, cakes, cinnamon buns, chips, crackers, doughnuts, muffins, piecrusts, many types of popcorn, and shortening.

marily those fats in your diet, they will not be easily stored on your body as fat, and this will ensure that the body has what it needs to construct the best lean muscles ever.

There are three omega fats: omega-3, omega-6, and omega-9. Which is the best? Your goal is to select items that are the *richest in omega-3*. Why? Omega-3 is the least-saturated fat—the most pliable and nonsolid. That means omega-3 fat is the body's top choice for maintaining everything from healthy cells to brain function to helping you restore lean muscle tissue. In fact, your body uses omega-3 fats for so many different functions that there isn't much left over to store in or on your body. It's kind of a fat-free fat! Isn't that amazing?

Which is my top omega-3 pick? *Flaxseed oil.* It is truly the best choice because it is the *richest source* of omega-3 fats. The oil is made by cold-pressing thousands of flaxseeds (also known as linseeds) to extract the oil. You can use the liquid form directly on your foods, and this is where the flavor and fun start. Think of it as a great flavor-enhancing condiment you can use with all your meals. Keep your portions to about 1 teaspoon per meal. I eat it on my toast at breakfast, I put it on my salad at lunch (see my salad dressing recipe on page 202), and at dinner I drizzle it over my steamed vegetables. Liquid flaxseed oil can be found in all health-food stores. And for those of you who travel or just don't care for the flavor, you can get flaxseed oil in capsule form, too. See the resources section for my favorite source of flaxseed oil.

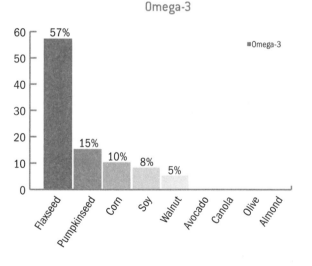

Water

Water is the one extra nutrient you need to take advantage of every day. It's the absolute essential beverage when you're trying to build lean muscle and burn fat. It's refreshing, filling, and calorie-free. When you don't get enough water, you feel sluggish, tired, and your muscles become tight and less metabolically active. In fact, dehydration even slows down your muscles' healing process after exercise! You might even feel hungry—the body sometimes misinterprets the signal for thirst as hunger—and overeat. It's vital to make sure that you drink enough water.

I suggest that you drink at least half of your body weight (in pounds) of water (in ounces) every day. That means, if you weigh 170 pounds, you should drink 85 ounces or about ten and a half 8-ounce glasses of water every day. It sounds like a lot, but it really isn't that hard. **The secret is to spread your drinking throughout the day and *make the water taste great.***

If you don't like to drink plain water, try and mix it up a bit with something that has flavor. I like Propel® Fit Water™ because it comes in great flavors (my favorite is lemonade), it's low in calories, and it's even a good source of vitamins C and B.

Yummy Recipes

In the back of this book you will find a week's worth of my best 12-Second Sequence™ recipes that can be made quickly and easily, allowing you to eat our 40/40/20 way.

Quick Home Cooking and Eating Out

Eating right on this plan is simple, whether you cook your own meals or eat out at restaurants. Here's how it works. Remember, if you weigh under 150 pounds, eat 3 ounces of protein at every meal; if you weigh over 150 pounds, eat 5 ounces of protein. For breakfast, I like to eat 3 scrambled eggs with two 1-ounce slices of turkey, ⅛ of an avocado, in a whole wheat tortilla and then have an apple for dessert. Yummy! This is what I do each morning. For lunch, you can eat 3 to 5 ounces of lean protein like a chicken or turkey breast, ½ cup of a whole wheat starchy carbohydrate like brown rice, and a big green salad with 1 teaspoon of my Lemon Flax Vinaigrette. Only at dinner will you *replace the starchy carbs like bread or rice with nonstarchy carbs like steamed vegetables*. For example, you might have 3 to 5 ounces of a grilled steak, a double serving of steamed broccoli, and a green salad with 1 teaspoon vinaigrette. Remember that vegetables are also carbs, but they're so high in fiber and water and so low in calories that your body doesn't store them as fat. Remember these guidelines when you're dining out, whether you're eating Mexican, Chinese, or Italian, so you can make sure that you're eating on plan wherever you are.

FREE DAY

I know that the idea of committing to a specific eating plan for an entire eight weeks makes some of you a little nervous. How can you possibly go eight weeks without your favorite ice cream or pizza? Well, I have some great news for you—you don't have to! I've built into the 12-Second Sequence™ an amazing day each week called your free day. Your free day is exactly that—it's a day that you can take each week to eat whatever you want. Really— whatever you want!

You may think that's impossible. How can I have a free day and still lose weight? Well, studies have shown that if you eat double the amount of calories you normally eat in one day, you will actually speed up your metabolism by 9 percent for the following 24 hours. That doesn't mean you get to double the number of calories you're eating on the other days; it just gives you complete freedom with your food choices for one day. I believe deprivation will only lead to bingeing, so this will allow you a small break to make sure you don't feel deprived of your favorite things.

I recommend picking the same day each week for your free day. I know I love to have Fridays for my free day because I like to have a great lunch with my team at my office and then take my wife and boys out to a nice dinner. Or maybe I want to go meet some friends out for a drink. The point is, try to pick a day that will work for you every week, whichever one it is.

There's only one catch to having a free day—it means no cheating on the other days of the week! But I think you're going to be surprised at how you feel after your free day. Because you are being so good to your body every other day of the week, you will be amazed at how lethargic and unhealthy you'll feel. In fact, I bet after a few free days, you will actually cut back just to a free meal or even just a small dessert or glass of wine. Once you realize the amazing power and energy you have when you're fueling your body with the right foods, you won't want to feel any other way—trust me.

Now, there may be some of you who don't need a free day or feel that maybe it will allow you to get off course too much; don't worry—this free day is completely optional. If you want to remain committed to the eating plan every day of the eight weeks, then that's great! In fact, you may even see accelerated results. The best thing is, it's up to you—the 12-Second Sequence™ is made to work for everyone, so customize it to fit your own lifestyle and goals.

START TODAY!

To help you track your meals and stick with the eating plan, I've included an Eating Planner in the resources section at the back of the book (see sample on page 39). It has space for your meals, snacks, water, and supplements. It also has time slots so you are sure to eat every three hours. It's easy to forget when to eat or whether you've had enough water for the day. Use this log to make sure that you stick to your eating plan and to your three-hour eating times. Remember, you can find this planner along with your Workout Logs in the *12-Second Sequence™ Journal* and on

12second.com. You can also find online the 7-Day Grid, which allows you to monitor your eating *and* your workouts with one handy sheet. Log on to the website today to print out your logs and get started!

Remember, it's critical to stick with a smart eating plan to get the most from your fitness routine, *so begin this plan at the time of your two-week Quick-Start phase.* Commit to eating right for the first two weeks, and when the advanced phase starts, you will be a true pro. You're going to see such *amazing* results that you'll never go back to your old eating habits.

EATING PLANNER (SAMPLE)

This plan will ensure leaner muscle and a higher metabolism.

Breakfast>time 7:30   Description

○	PROTEIN* (3–5oz/40g)	smoked salmon
○	CARBS (½ cup or 1 slice of bread)	whole-grain bread
○	FRUIT (1 cup)	cantaloupe
○	FAT (1 teaspoon)	1 tsp. flax oil on toast

Snack>time 10:30   Description

○	WHEY PROTEIN SHAKE (1 scoop)	Jorge's Packs choc. shake

Jorge recommends Jorge's Packs™ for your protein drinks. **>** See list of other recommended snacks at the back.

Lunch>time 1:30   Description

○	PROTEIN* (3–5oz/40g)	turkey burger
○	CARBS (½ cup or 1 slice of bread)	whole-grain bun
○	VEGGIES** (2 cups)	mixed greens
○	FAT (1 teaspoon)	flax dressing

Snack>time 4:30   Description

○	WHEY PROTEIN SHAKE (1 scoop)	Jorge's Packs vanilla shake

Dinner>time 7:30   Description

○	PROTEIN* (3–5oz/40g)	chicken breast
○	VEGGIES** (2–4 cups)	broccoli florets
○	FAT (1 teaspoon)	olive oil

Snack>time 10:30   Description

○	WHEY PROTEIN SHAKE (1 scoop)	Jorge's Packs choc. shake

*If you weigh under 150 pounds, eat 3 ounces of protein at every meal; if you weigh over 150 pounds, eat 5 ounces of protein.

**Veggies = nonstarchy vegetables.

Water (eight 8-oz cups) ● ● ● ● ● ● ● ○

Multivitamin ●

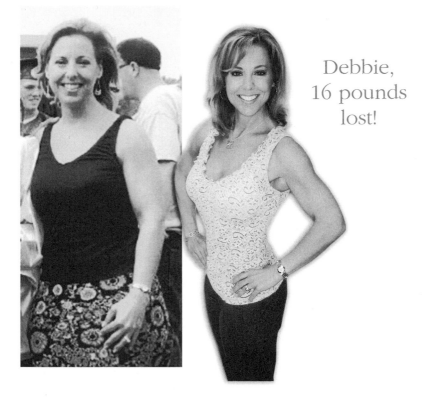

Debbie, 16 pounds lost!

"In the past year, I noticed that my small waist was getting bigger and I was losing my overall muscle tone. I knew I had to do something. And then I found Jorge's 12-Second Sequence™ program.

"After just 8 weeks, I once again have my small waist, and my overall muscle tone has improved significantly. The bonus is that I also feel energetic and young! This program enables excellent physical health, which ultimately promotes excellent psychological health—a perfect balance."

DEBBIE'S SECRETS TO SUCCESS

· If you deviate from the program at all, get right back on track—do not let one slip turn into two or more.
· Absolutely do your cardio every morning upon rising and before eating!
· Plan, plan, plan! Know in advance what you will need to prepare in order to fit the program into your day-to-day schedule.

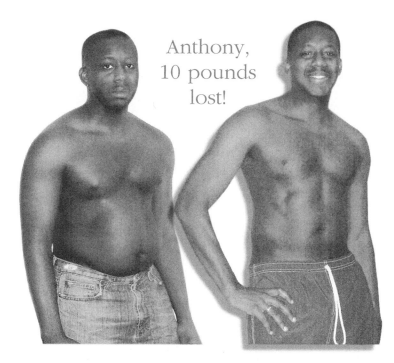

Anthony,
10 pounds
lost!

12
SECOND
STAR

**ANTHONY
BENNETT**

Age: 39
Height: 5'6"
Lost: 10 pounds

"Thanks to the 12-Second Sequence™, life is great! This program is perfect for the busy parent—just 20 minutes, twice a week. I have more energy, I feel I am in control of my life, and I look awesome. I've lost 10 pounds and 4 percent body fat after seven weeks.

"After being depressed for many years, this program has given me a passion to follow my dreams and goals. In order to celebrate my upcoming fortieth birthday, I bought a bike to ride and train for the 26-mile L.A. Acura Bike Tour—I'm now up for the challenge and ready to live life to the fullest. Thanks, Jorge!"

ANTHONY'S SECRETS TO SUCCESS

· Mineral water with a splash of lemon goes great with any meal.
· Rewrite your Success Contract at the beginning of each week.
· When cravings are getting the best of you, take a deep breath and imagine what your life would be like at your goal weight.

HOW TO CONQUER THE NIGHT 5

Before the 12-Second Sequence™, I was never able to stick to a plan. But with Jorge's help my emotional fitness became stronger. I feel great now; strong and proud. People are noticing that I've changed. I want to tell everyone about how the program changed my life!

—JANET KEITH, *12-Second Star, lost 18 pounds*

In my experience, the time you're most likely to be tempted to sabotage all your hard work by overeating is at night. So I created this chapter to empower you emotionally. I want you to build your inner strength, so you have *control* of your eating at night, and so that you have the motivation never to skip a workout during your 8-Week Challenge. It will help build the kind of discipline that comes from having true **inner strength.** Most people never develop that. All they have is a New Year's resolution that stays strong for about a week before they lose their focus. That will not help you achieve your goals. That is not good enough. You need a more sophisticated system to better inspire you to stick to your plan and make it *automatic*.

Sound good? Let's get started.

KNOW YOUR EXACT GOALS

The very first thing you must do right now is *define* on paper what your exact goals are. You see, if you don't have a clear vision of what you want to accomplish with this program, you will most likely fail in the long term. Yes, that's a big statement to make, but I know it's the truth. I have seen so many successful clients that I know the road map to success. And if you don't have a strong enough vision you will fail. That is why right now we are going to define precisely what your goals will be. You will need three goals. First of all, what do you want to accomplish in the first two weeks? Next, think about what you want to have accomplished at the end of the 8-Week Challenge. Finally, you must have what I call a lifetime goal. Reviewing these three goals each morning will ignite your drive throughout the next few weeks. Place your Success Contract on your refrigerator door to keep you on track.

What can you realistically expect of yourself? Most people drop one to two sizes in their waist within the first two weeks. By the end of the 8-Week Challenge, you could lose 30 pounds or more! Those are excellent and realistic outcomes for your first two goals. For your lifetime goal, you want to focus on a *health*-related objective. Keeping your waist below 35 inches if you're a man and 32.5 inches if you're a woman is one of the most important things you can do to avoid life-threatening diseases like diabetes, heart disease, and even certain cancers.

In the column on the right is the line "I Want to Feel." I'm including this because I think so many fitness programs neglect to address an amazing outcome of exercise, which is how it makes you *feel*. So I want you to think about how you want to feel throughout the 8-Week Challenge and how you want to feel when you complete it. Do you want to feel confident? Strong? Empowered? Energetic? I know it might sound corny, but I promise you, giving yourself a feeling to strive for will give you that extra drive and focus you need. Make sure you pick a word that has nothing to do with weight or your body. I want you to commit to a *feeling* because that feeling is what's going to transform your life.

Think about these goals as a cake. Next, I want you to add the frosting on the cake. It will sweeten and strengthen your motivation even more. **I want you to create a visual Success Line.** What is this? Well, I strongly believe that nothing is as powerful as our own history to remind us of things we have overcome and accomplished. The challenge is that many times we forget what we have already accomplished and, mistakenly, we feel weak and powerless.

So here is what I want you to do. I want you to write down the top four proudest moments in your life. It can be anything: finishing high school, getting your first job, the birth of your child, or a demonstration of your artistic talent. It doesn't matter what the moments are; all that matters is that you write down four events that truly remind you that you *can do it*. These kind of reminders are critical helpers, particularly when you post them in places where you'll see them often, like the refrigerator. That way, when you walk by your Success Line at night on the way to the ice cream, you'll stay on course instead.

SUCCESS CONTRACT

Photocopy and place on the refrigerator, in the pantry, or at your bedside.

Today's date: _____

My 2-Week Goal:

I Want to Feel:

My Goal for the 8-Week Challenge:

My Lifetime Goal:

Signature: _____

MY SUCCESS LINE

Photocopy and place on the refrigerator, in the pantry, or at your bedside.

1st event	2nd event	3rd event	4th event	5th event	6th event
				Committing to the 12-Second Sequence™ 8-Week Challenge today! My current weight: _____ My current size: _____	Finishing the 12-Second Sequence™ 8-Week Challenge! My new weight: _____ My new size: _____
Insert Photo	Insert Photo	Insert Photo	Insert Photo	Insert Photo	Insert Photo
				Take before photo now and place it here.	Visit 12second. com and create a virtual image of what you'll look like when you reach your goal.

If you can, add a photo of each meaningful event. It will magnify the emotional impact that these reminders have and increase your motivation. This will be a second layer of frosting, and very important to sweetening your success. Once completed, photocopy and place your Success Line in your kitchen, your bedroom, and even on your bathroom mirror.

TRACKING YOUR SUCCESS

As you begin your workouts and eating plan, I want you to keep a log of your daily results. There are three logs in the back of this book, two for your workouts and one for your eating. You should photocopy them and use them each day to keep on track. They also have space for writing down additional notes to yourself. *Think of these logs as additional motivational tools that will keep you aware of what you're doing and what you have done.* After the 8-Week Challenge, looking back on these will help keep you motivated to continue the program. They will be your personal blueprints to your best and healthiest body ever.

If you want a great online version of our log system, visit 12second.com. And if you want our printed version for the full eight weeks, then make sure to pick up a copy of our companion journal available at bookstores everywhere and on our website.

THE POWER OF PEOPLE

There's one last secret I want to share with you that will help you conquer the night and keep your motivation super-high throughout the whole eight weeks—*the power of people*. What do I mean? Well, having the support of people who care about your success is probably the number one secret of my most successful clients.

You see, *you become who you are with*. That is a powerful statement, and it means that the peo-

ple around you indirectly affect who you become in life. If you have a great circle of friends, then you will do great. But if you have a negative circle or no circle, then the odds are against you. What can you do? Well, that is why I created our online club at 12second.com. It is a virtual community and support center where you can go 24 hours a day to meet other people who are on the plan. Every day you can connect with thousands of people going through the same triumphs and frustrations that you are. You can discuss your experiences and make wonderful new friends. It's a place where you can create accountability buddies, as well as e-mail and phone buddies. Bottom line: It can be the place that empowers you each day during the 8-Week Challenge. I am also there hosting daily coaching sessions. I hope to see you there and have you join our online family!

SECOND
STAR

JANET KEITH

Age: 51
Height: 5'6"
Lost: 16 pounds

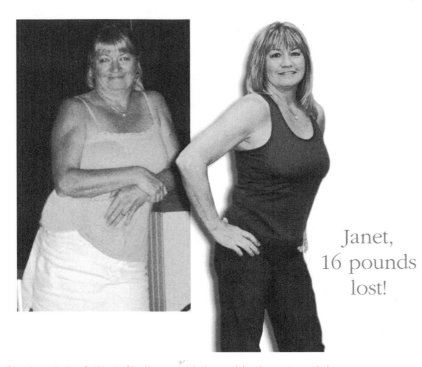

Janet,
16 pounds
lost!

"Before I took the 8-Week Challenge with Jorge, I had no strength in my arms or abs. I would go back and forth with different exercise plans and I was never able to stick with one. I needed help! I never had enough energy to try outdoor activities, and I hated the way my clothes fit and how I felt about myself.

"Now I have so much energy from doing the 12-Second Sequence™ that my co-workers are telling me I talk too much! I am motivated to go places and do things instead of just sitting around in front of the TV. I have a shape—and that's something I haven't seen for years. I got all this from a simple workout that was so easy to work into my life—and stick to!

"I feel great, strong, and proud of myself now. People are noticing that I have changed, and I want to tell everyone about the 12-Second Sequence™!"

JANET'S SECRETS TO SUCCESS

· Planning meals ahead of time.
· Quiet time to exercise with no interruptions.
· Visualizing the "new" me.

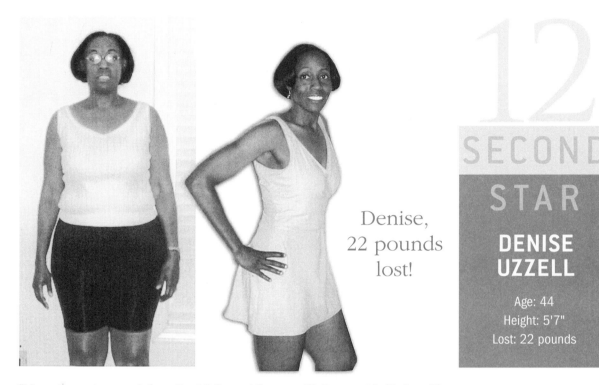

Denise, 22 pounds lost!

"I have learned so much from the 12-Second Sequence™. I've spent half of my life going from one diet to another. I'd lose the weight then I'd wonder how I could keep it off once I started eating regular food again.

"This time I've learned how to eat healthfully by eating regular foods instead of processed foods. I made a lifestyle change instead of just dieting. I am forty-four years old with an eight-year-old son. Failure was not an option for me. I've learned that eating right is only one part of the equation. Working out is just as important.

"To sum it up, when I look good, I feel good. Right now, I feel GREAT and look forward to my next challenge."

DENISE'S SECRETS FOR SUCCESS

- · Do the morning cardio! Doing cardio keeps the pounds melting off and keeps you energized.
- · Have something to motivate you, a goal or reward, or possibly a trip.
- · Think about how your being healthy helps motivate others around you, like your friends and family.

GET READY TO START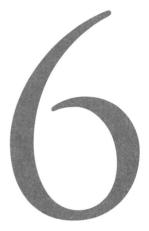

Never before have I lost so many inches so quickly. It's been incredible! **I have lost a total of 18 inches off my body.** My clothes fit differently and people have really noticed the changes.
—CHRISTINE RIVERA, *12-Second Star, lost 20 pounds*

T here are two simple phases of the 12-Second Sequence™ that you will follow over the next eight weeks. The two phases are designed to work together, and it's important for you to follow the phases to see the absolute maximum results.

Quick-Start Phase

This phase is designed to get you going fast. The workouts require absolutely *no* gym and can be done easily at your home. After the first week your workouts will become progressively more intense, which will get you ready for the advanced phase.

The first two weeks require just a few simple tools: **a set of dumbbells, a Swiss ball, and a mat.** You can find this equipment at any sporting goods store or on our website. My favorite brand is one called GoFit.™ You can find more information about GoFit™ products in the resources section.

Now, if you have a gym membership then you of course can do all the Quick-Start workouts there. Nothing wrong with that at all. But either way, there's no excuse not to get started!

A "No-Excuses" Week 1

The equipment you need to start the 12-Second Sequence™ is minimal—a Swiss ball, a mat, and a set of dumbbells. However, if you don't have these items and want to start the program today, well, believe it or not, you can! In the resources section, you'll find an on-the-go, weight-free workout that will let you get started without any special equipment. All you need is a chair and a mat or towel. You create all the resistance you need with your own body weight. This workout is not only perfect to get you started on the program, but it's also great for when you're traveling or in your office at work. You'll work your entire body in one 20-minute workout. To get started, do this circuit two times in your first week, ideally on Monday and Thursday. Then, get ready to step up the intensity and begin with Week 1!

Advanced Phase

Once you complete the Quick-Start Phase, you will move immediately to the Advanced Phase. This doesn't mean you have to be an Olympic athlete to do these exercises, it just means we're going to continue to challenge your body. Remember, that's what will transform your lean muscle. The 12-Second Sequence™ is designed to truly change your body, which is why we have to introduce you progressively to new exercises that create the best results possible.

The first two weeks of the Advanced Phase will incorporate many new moves and will still require your dumbbells, Swiss ball, and mat. You can also continue to work out in your own home if that's where you're most comfortable. *But things will change when we start week 5.* **To progressively challenge your muscles best, you will need to start using a "functional trainer" (FT) cable machine when you reach week 5.**

Incorporating an FT cable machine will take your workout to the next level. Why? Nothing else is as effective. *An FT cable machine gives you the balance and stability of free weights, yet still provides a consistent amount of resistance like a traditional machine.* Traditional non-FT machines allow for constant resistance on your muscles, but because they follow a "track motion," they don't fully engage your stabilizer muscles. And that means that you aren't maximizing your workout. And remember, that's our goal here—to create the *challenge* that will best sculpt and shape your gorgeous lean muscle. Bottom line—for maximum results, do everything you can to get access to an FT cable machine.

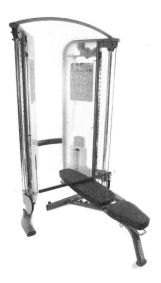

Where can you find an FT cable machine? Well, you have two options: the first is to purchase one for your home. In my opinion there truly is no better investment for your health. No fancy car is going to improve the length and quality of your life as much as investing in your health and fitness. I recommend a product called Precor® S3.23. Look in the resources section for more information.

The second option is to go to a gym. All gyms will have an FT cable machine or something similar. If you don't see a machine that resembles the one pictured in this book, talk to one of your gym's employees, and they'll direct you to the appropriate equipment. What do you do if you don't belong to a gym? I have great news: The folks at Bally® Total Fitness have agreed to offer a free 12-Second Sequence™ class when you download the pass from 12second.com. Turn to the resources section for more information on Bally®. And if you absolutely can't get to the gym, check out another option in chapter 10.

I understand that some people may have injuries or other conditions that may make it difficult to complete some of the moves. That's why you'll see a "Backup move" option for certain exercises. Remember, the pictured move is ideal, but you can still get good results if you complete the backup move instead.

HOW IT'S DONE

In chapter 3, you learned how the 12-Second Sequence™ works your body out in two groups—primary muscles and secondary muscles—and that you're going to be doing three circuits each day that target those specific parts of your body. Remember, each circuit is four exercises, and you do four reps of each exercise. So when you start day 1 with a lunge for your legs, you're going to do four lunges with the powerful 12-Second Sequence™ count and then move quickly into your next exercise. When you add it up, each circuit is actually about six minutes, so your workout for the day is only 18 minutes long, but I included a little time for you to transition to the next exercise. So there you go—20 minutes, twice a week.

THE BEST DAYS

Now, you could do your two weekly workouts on any two days of the week that work best for you, but there is one essential requirement. If you really want to see the best results, you need to allow your body two days of rest between workouts. If you do the workouts too close together, you will not be sufficiently rested and your muscles will not be fully recovered. **My official recommendation is to do the workouts on Mondays and Thursdays.** My most successful clients love starting the week off with a great workout and then getting the second one in before the weekend. But you can do them whenever it's best for you—just remember to let your body rest in between. Use the 8-Week Workout Chart (opposite) to check off your workouts as you perform them.

Finally, I need to share with you my *four technique secrets:* form, counting, breathing, and intensity. They are easy to understand, but getting these four things right is going to guarantee maximum results for you.

WHY FORM IS IMPORTANT

When you perform the exercises the right way, you concentrate the stress on the muscle you're working. When you do a biceps curl, for example, you want the full weight of the dumbbell or cable on *only* your biceps. If you compromise your form, you allow other muscle groups like your shoulders or your back to support the weight. **Bad form, therefore, cheats you out of a truly effective workout**—and could even lead to debilitating injuries that keep you from working out for weeks!

In chapter 7 you will see that each exercise has two pictures of me demonstrating the move (some have three for special grips and other specific instructions) and then a brief description of how to do it. **It's important for you to read the descriptions!** You will see key tips like "keep your back straight," or "keep your elbows close to your body throughout the exercise," that will be essential to your success. Think of these descriptions as recipes. You wouldn't make lasagna for the first time without reading the recipe, right? So if you are truly committed to creating your best body, you can't leave any key ingredients out! As you go through the workouts, read the descriptions in chapters 7 and 8 for the exact details, but here are some general tips for success.

Because our goal with the 12-Second Sequence™ is to work as efficiently as possible, I want you to do a few things in preparation. Start by reviewing the circuits before you do the workout for the day. Look at each one and do a quick practice run to familiarize yourself with the movement and see where your maximum tension point (MTP) is going to be. That way, when you start your chair dip, for example, you'll know exactly where the 2-second hold will

8-WEEK WORKOUT CHART

Start>date ___1/7___   Finish>date ___2/28___

	Monday	Tuesday	Wednesday	Thursday	Friday	Saturday	Sunday
WEEK 1	DAY 1 ~~X~~ PRIMARY WORKOUT 1/7	DAY 2 ~~X~~ DAY OFF	DAY 3 ~~X~~ DAY OFF	DAY 4 ~~X~~ SECONDARY WORKOUT 1/10	DAY 5 ~~X~~ DAY OFF	DAY 6 ~~X~~ DAY OFF	DAY 7 ~~X~~ DAY OFF
WEEK 2	DAY 8 ~~X~~ PRIMARY WORKOUT 1/14	DAY 9 ~~X~~ DAY OFF	DAY 10 ~~X~~ DAY OFF	DAY 11 ~~X~~ SECONDARY WORKOUT 1/17	DAY 12 ~~X~~ DAY OFF	DAY 13 ~~X~~ DAY OFF	DAY 14 ~~X~~ DAY OFF
WEEK 3	DAY 15 ~~X~~ PRIMARY WORKOUT 1/21	DAY 16 ~~X~~ DAY OFF	DAY 17 ~~X~~ DAY OFF	DAY 18 ~~X~~ SECONDARY WORKOUT 1/24	DAY 19 ~~X~~ DAY OFF	DAY 20 ~~X~~ DAY OFF	DAY 21 ~~X~~ DAY OFF
WEEK 4	DAY 22 ~~X~~ PRIMARY WORKOUT 1/28	DAY 23 ~~X~~ DAY OFF	DAY 24 ~~X~~ DAY OFF	DAY 25 ~~X~~ SECONDARY WORKOUT 1/31	DAY 26 ~~X~~ DAY OFF	DAY 27 ~~X~~ DAY OFF	DAY 28 ~~X~~ DAY OFF
WEEK 5	DAY 29 ~~X~~ PRIMARY WORKOUT 2/4	DAY 30 ~~X~~ DAY OFF	DAY 31 ~~X~~ DAY OFF	DAY 32 ~~X~~ SECONDARY WORKOUT 2/7	DAY 33 ~~X~~ DAY OFF	DAY 34 DAY OFF	DAY 35 DAY OFF
WEEK 6	DAY 36 PRIMARY WORKOUT 2/11	DAY 37 DAY OFF	DAY 38 DAY OFF	DAY 39 SECONDARY WORKOUT 2/14	DAY 40 DAY OFF	DAY 41 DAY OFF	DAY 42 DAY OFF
WEEK 7	DAY 43 PRIMARY WORKOUT 2/18	DAY 44 DAY OFF	DAY 45 DAY OFF	DAY 46 SECONDARY WORKOUT 2/21	DAY 47 DAY OFF	DAY 48 DAY OFF	DAY 49 DAY OFF
WEEK 8	DAY 50 PRIMARY WORKOUT 2/25	DAY 51 DAY OFF	DAY 52 DAY OFF	DAY 53 SECONDARY WORKOUT 2/28	DAY 54 DAY OFF	DAY 55 DAY OFF	DAY 56 SUCCESS!

*Please photocopy and place on your refrigerator. As you complete your workouts, cross off the days so you can see your success!

work best for you. Remember, the circuit element of this workout will keep your heart rate up, so the better you know the movements before you start, the quicker you can move through them. Even though I've included some transition time between exercises, the more familiar you are with what comes next, the better cardio effect you will get from the workouts. Don't get frustrated if you feel that the right form comes slowly to you at first—it will get easier and easier every time you do it!

One more thing: Don't forget your morning cardio! Remember to take a brisk 20-minute walk every morning before breakfast. As I stated in chapter 3, walking in the morning will accelerate your fat burning and get you to your goal weight in even less time. Refer to chapter 3 if you need to refresh yourself on the benefits of walking.

You've got all the tools you need to get started. I know you're ready to begin the program that will change your life and body forever.

COUNTING

I know you learned about how the 12-Second Sequence™ works in chapter 3, but I want to remind you just how essential counting is going to be to your success. Remember, you start with a 10-second positive motion, hold for 2 seconds at the MTP, and return to your starting position through another count of 10 seconds. This unique, revolutionary *timing* is what is going to transform your body into a lean, toned, fat-burning machine!

If you want a neat tool to help you get the timing down, one of my clients shared with me the idea of using a metronome. It was originally created to help musicians maintain tempo, but a lot of my clients found that it was perfect for helping them count their 12 seconds accurately. You can find metronomes at music equipment stores or at 12second.com.

Whatever counting method you use, it's important to stick to the 10-second motions and 2-second hold at the MTP. If you move faster, you'll increase your momentum and minimize the impact on your muscle. Don't cheat yourself! As you finish one rep, move right into your next one until you complete the recommended number of reps. When you keep the movement continuous throughout the whole set, you will be amazed at how effectively you create that muscle burn in such a short time.

BREATHING

When it comes to breathing, I have found that some of my clients have a tendency to hold their breath while exercising or sometimes even hyperventilate. Doing either of these doesn't allow the proper amount of oxygen to be delivered throughout the body. Oxygen is crucial when it comes to exercise. It combines with glycogen and fat to produce energy and give you the strength to continue working out. Due to the unique nature of the 12-Second Sequence™, I recommend a technique known as feathered breathing. Feathered breathing is a method of controlled breathing for when oxygen uptake is needed over a sustained period of exertion. This is a steady, rhythmic breathing pattern that will prevent you from holding your breath or hyperventilating. The technique is very simple and with a little practice you will master it in no time. You simply take a deep breath in just before you begin your exercise, and then in a controlled pattern exhale with short bursts. When your lungs have emptied, you will take another deep breath in and continue to exhale with short breaths throughout the exercise. Continue the method throughout the entire set. Visit 12second.com for a free demo of our feathered breathing technique.

INTENSITY

Intensity is a crucial element of your 12-Second Sequence™ workout. Since you're only doing four reps total for most of the exercises, it's important to make those reps really count. Remember, this workout is only 20 minutes, twice a week. Giving your best effort during those minutes will make all the difference in your results. Here are some pointers on how to create the ideal intensity for *your* workout.

Pick the *right* weight, because this will cause muscle fatigue by the fourth rep. You can use three sets of dumbbells—5-, 10-, and 15-pound—or an all-in-one dumbbell system.

Because keeping the intensity up is key, you've got to make sure you are using the right amount of weight for each exercise. **Here is the test:** If you can lift the weight for more than four reps, the weight you are using is not heavy enough. And if you can only complete two or three reps, then—you can probably guess this—the weight is too heavy! It's a very simple formula, but it's essential that you maximize the effect of every single rep—keeping the right intensity is absolutely crucial to getting the most out of the plan. Again, don't cheat yourself out of the best workout because you will cheat yourself out of seeing the best *results* possible— and that's why you're here, right? To develop the shapely, lean muscle that burns body fat 24 hours a day.

Refer back to this chapter whenever you need to refresh your memory on proper form, breathing, counting, or level of intensity. The tools I've outlined in this chapter will allow you to get the most out of the time you spend exercising. Not only that, but doing each exercise with the right form will create the most effective and safe workout.

You are now ready to get started with the Quick-Start Phase. Let's do it!

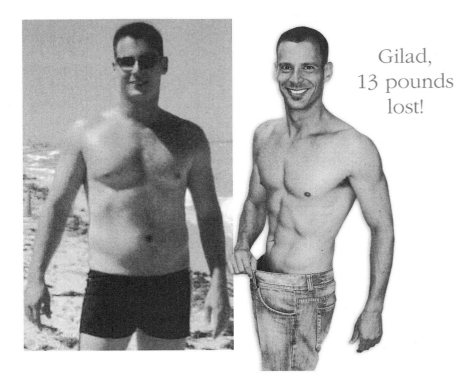

12 SECOND STAR

GILAD BARASH

Age: 35
Height: 5'8"
Lost: 13 pounds

Gilad,
13 pounds
lost!

"I have always led a pretty sedentary lifestyle. I tried to make physical fitness a priority, but school and then work took up most of my time. I went through phases of bulking up and slimming down and even tried working with trainers. This time, however, I wanted to try something different. I wanted to lose the 10 pounds that I've never been able to lose.

"The 12-Second Sequence™ came at just the right time. The program gave me the direction and the tools that, coupled with dedication, helped me get rid of those pesky 10 pounds—plus a few more! And I am confident that this program has given me the tools to maintain these fantastic results."

GILAD'S SECRETS TO SUCCESS

· Seeing results was the single greatest motivator I had, and it made me want to continue and see more results.
· Incorporate a cheat meal into your week to resist binges and to stay motivated.

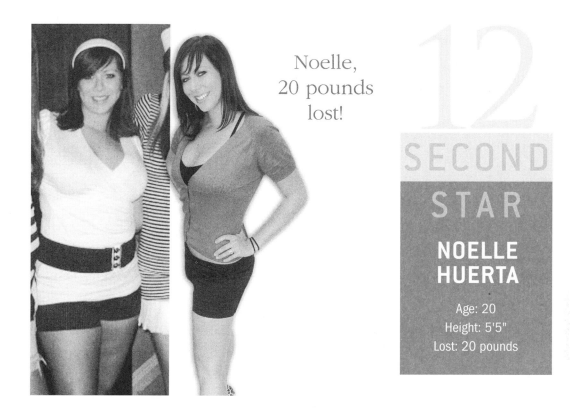

Noelle,
20 pounds
lost!

12 SECOND STAR

NOELLE HUERTA

Age: 20
Height: 5'5"
Lost: 20 pounds

"With the combination of little exercise, a poor diet, and a new environment after starting college, I gained the 'freshman fifteen' and more. By the end of my freshman year I was over 150 pounds, something that I had never been. When I began the 12-Second Sequence™, I was extremely motivated because I knew I could do it and see results.

"Although I have completed 8 weeks, it doesn't mean that I will stop the program. It is now how I live my life. I have learned to create a routine that gets diet and exercise into my crazy and busy life. I have seen my confidence increase so much and I can't wait to see even more results!"

NOELLE'S SECRETS TO SUCCESS

· Don't give up! If you don't see results right away, don't feel down.
· Plan your meals ahead of time, so you have no excuse not to eat every 3 hours.
· Do the morning cardio—it really works!

QUICK-START PHASE

7

WEEKS 1 TO 2

LEGS

EXERCISE A

Beginner Squat

Stand between two sturdy chairs with your feet shoulder-width apart. Feather your breathing as you slowly squat through a count of 10 seconds—keeping your back straight, abs tight, and chest up. Hold for 2 seconds at the MTP. Return to starting position through a count of 10 seconds. Without resting, repeat three times. (Note: Be sure to use the chairs only for balance, not to hold your weight.)

1

2

BACK

EXERCISE B

Pullover on Swiss Ball

Grasp a dumbbell using the diamond grip. Lie on the ball with your head and neck supported. Keep your hips up and abs tight throughout the exercise. Extend the weight over your chest with a slight bend in the elbows. Feather your breathing as you lower the weight down behind your head through a count of 10 seconds. Hold for 2 seconds at the MTP. Raise the weight back to starting point through a count of 10 seconds. Without resting, repeat three times. (Note: How far you can stretch your arms back will determine your MTP.)

DIAMOND GRIP

1

2

KEY: MTP: maximum tension point. **Feather your breathing:** Inhale deeply and exhale in short bursts.
Timing: Each exercise should take 90 seconds, and each circuit should take 6 minutes.

CHEST

EXERCISE C

Incline Press on Swiss Ball

Hold a pair of dumbbells and lie on the ball so that your head and neck are supported. Allow your hips to drop almost to the ground. Press the weights up and together, with a slight bend in the elbows so that the upper chest is targeted. Feather your breathing as you lower the weights down through a count of 10 seconds. Hold for 2 seconds at the MTP. Press the dumbbells up to starting point through a count of 10 seconds. Without resting, repeat three times.

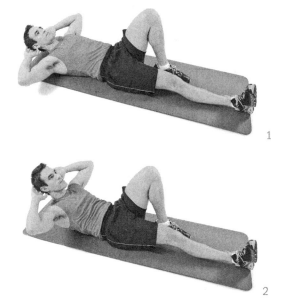

1

2

ABS

EXERCISE D

Curl-up Crunch

Lie flat on a mat. Place your hands behind your head to support your neck. Bend one knee, but keep your other leg straight. Feather your breathing as you curl up and crunch toward your knees through a count of 10 seconds. Hold and squeeze for 2 seconds at the MTP. Return back to starting point through a count of 10 seconds. Without resting, repeat once more. Switch legs and complete 2 more reps, for a total of 4.

1

2

LEGS

EXERCISE A

Swiss Ball Squat

Place the ball against a wall and position yourself with the ball supporting your lower back. Stand with your feet hip-width apart, about 1 foot from the wall. Cross your arms in front of your shoulders. Feather your breathing as you squat through a count of 10 to about a 90-degree angle. Hold at the MTP for 2 seconds, and then return to starting point through a count of 10 seconds. Without resting, repeat three times.

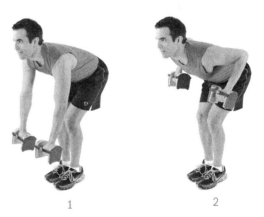

1   2

BACK

EXERCISE B

Bent-over Row (overhand grip)

Hold a pair of dumbbells, arms extended, palms facing back. Stand with your feet hip-width apart. Bend at the waist as if tying your shoes. Raise your head and chest to create a slight arch in the back. Bend your knees slightly. Feather your breathing as you pull the dumbbells up in a fluid rowing motion through a count of 10 seconds, keeping your elbows close to your body. Hold and squeeze your shoulder blades together at the MTP for 2 seconds. Lower your arms back to starting point through a count of 10. Without resting, repeat three times.

1   2

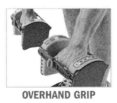

OVERHAND GRIP

KEY: **MTP:** maximum tension point. **Feather your breathing:** Inhale deeply and exhale in short bursts.
Timing: Each exercise should take 90 seconds, and each circuit should take 6 minutes.

CHEST

EXERCISE C

Push-up on Knees

Kneel on a mat on all fours, with your knees hip-width apart. Your hands should be slightly wider than shoulder-width apart and your fingers and wrists pointing forward. Feather your breathing as you lower your chest toward the floor through a count of 10 seconds. Hold for 2 seconds at the MTP. Push your body back to starting position through a count of 10 seconds, keeping your elbows slightly bent at the top of the move. Without resting, repeat three times.

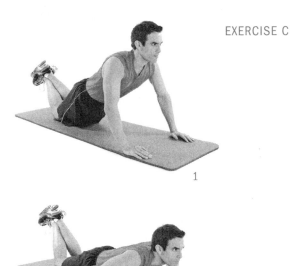

ABS

EXERCISE D

Chair Crunch

Sit on the front edge of a sturdy chair or workout bench. Reach your hands behind you and grab the sides of the chair. Extend your legs out and allow your upper body to recline back slightly. Feather your breathing as you slowly draw your knees in and up toward your chest through a count of 10 seconds. Hold and squeeze at MTP for 2 seconds. Return legs to starting point through a count of 10 seconds. Without resting, repeat three times.

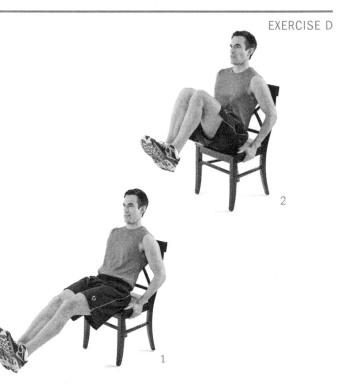

LEGS

Plié Squat

Hold one dumbbell with both hands and stand with your feet about twice shoulder-width apart, toes turned out to the sides aligning with your knees. Feather your breathing as you squat (as if you were sitting into a chair) through a count of 10 seconds. Hold for 2 seconds at the MTP. Push through your heels, returning to starting point through a count of 10. Without resting, repeat three times.

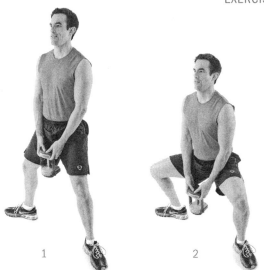

BACK

Hyperextension on Swiss Ball

Lie on the ball with your hips supported and your hands behind your head. Bend at the waist. Feather your breathing as you lift your upper body through a count of 10 seconds, using your lower back. Hold for 2 seconds at the MTP. Return to starting point through a count of 10 seconds. Without resting, repeat three times.

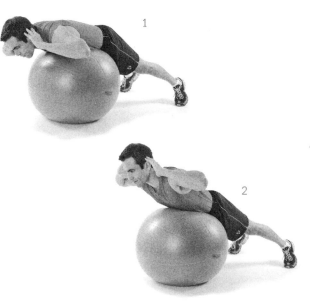

KEY: MTP: maximum tension point. **Feather your breathing:** Inhale deeply and exhale in short bursts.
Timing: Each exercise should take 90 seconds, and each circuit should take 6 minutes.

CHEST

Flat Dumbbell Fly on Swiss Ball

Hold a pair of dumbbells and lie on the ball with your head and neck supported. Extend the dumbbells over your chest, palms facing each other, elbows slightly bent. Feather your breathing as you lower the weights down and out through a count of 10 seconds. Hold for 2 seconds at the MTP, and then raise the weight back to starting point in a "bear hug" motion through a count of 10 seconds. Without resting, repeat three times.

ABS

Broomstick Twist

Stand with your legs about 3 feet apart. Place a broomstick across the back of your shoulders, grip with your hands, and twist your upper body to one side. With your chin up and abs squeezed tight, feather your breathing as you slowly twist to the other side through a count of 10 seconds. At the MTP of your twist, hold and squeeze for 2 seconds. Return to starting point through a count of 10. Without resting, repeat three times. (Note: If you can do more than 4 reps, you're not squeezing your abs hard enough throughout the exercise.)

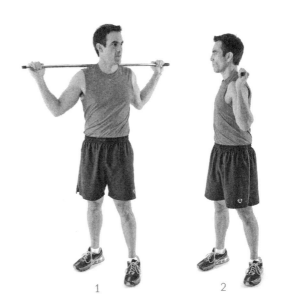

FINISH

START

SHOULDERS

EXERCISE A

Standing Shoulder Press

Hold a pair of dumbbells and stand with your feet slightly apart and knees slightly bent, your back straight, abs tight, and chin up. Extend the weights up and together directly over your head, palms facing forward. Feather your breathing as you lower the weights down through a count of 10 seconds. Hold for 2 seconds at the MTP (chin level). Press the dumbbells up to starting point through a count of 10 seconds. Without resting, repeat three times.

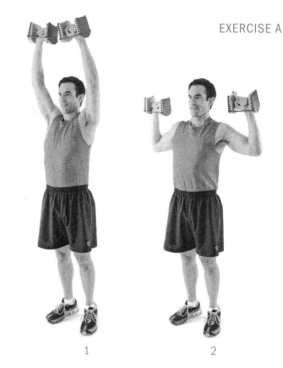

1   2

BICEPS

EXERCISE B

Standing Curl

Hold a pair of dumbbells and stand with your feet shoulder-width apart and your arms extended by your sides, with your palms facing forward and your knees slightly bent. Feather your breathing as you curl the dumbbells up through a count of 10 seconds to just past a 90-degree angle. Hold and squeeze for 2 seconds at the MTP. Keep your elbows tight against your body as you lower the weights to starting point through a count of 10 seconds. Without resting, repeat three times. (Note: Keep your elbows tight against your sides throughout the entire exercise.)

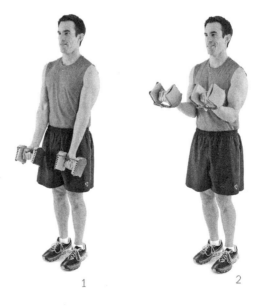

1   2

KEY: MTP: maximum tension point. **Feather your breathing:** Inhale deeply and exhale in short bursts. **Timing:** Each exercise should take 90 seconds, and each circuit should take 6 minutes.

TRICEPS

EXERCISE C

Chair Dip

Sit on the edge of a very sturdy chair or workout bench with your hands behind you and fingers forward, grasping the front edge of the chair. Flex your feet so that your weight is on your heels and slide yourself away from the chair. Feather your breathing as you lower yourself through a count of 10 seconds. Hold for 2 seconds at the MTP. Push yourself back up to starting point through a count of 10 seconds. Without resting, repeat three times. (Note: The MTP will depend on how flexible your shoulders are—about an inch above your most flexible point.)

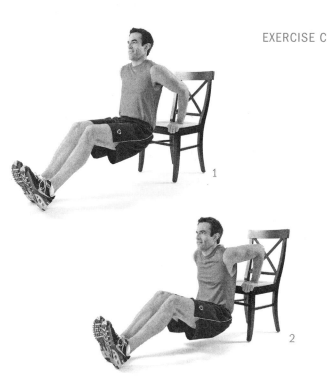

ABS

EXERCISE D

Toe Reach

Lie on your back. Cross your legs, flex your feet, and extend your legs into the air. With your arms extended and chin up, feather your breathing as you crunch up, reaching toward your toes through a count of 10 seconds. Hold and squeeze for 2 seconds at the MTP. Lower yourself back to starting position, keeping your shoulder blades from touching the ground, through a count of 10 seconds. Without resting, repeat three times.

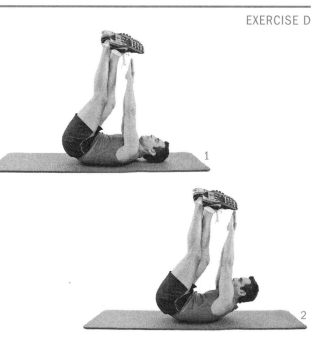

SHOULDERS

Standing Lateral Raise

Hold a pair of dumbbells and stand with your feet together, back straight, and abs tight. With your arms against your sides and elbows slightly bent, feather your breathing as you raise the weights up through a count of 10 seconds. Hold and squeeze at the MTP ("T" position) for 2 seconds. Lower weight to starting point through a count of 10 seconds. Without resting, repeat three times.

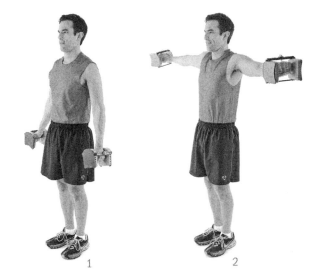

1   2

BICEPS

Side Curl on Swiss Ball

Hold a pair of dumbbells and sit on the ball. With your arms down against your sides, palms turned up, and elbows tight against your body, feather your breathing as you curl the weights up through a count of 10 seconds. Hold and squeeze for 2 seconds at the MTP. Lower the weights to starting point through a count of 10 seconds. Without resting, repeat three times.

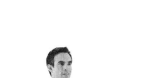

1   2

KEY: MTP: maximum tension point. **Feather your breathing:** Inhale deeply and exhale in short bursts.
Timing: Each exercise should take 90 seconds, and each circuit should take 6 minutes.

TRICEPS

EXERCISE C

Dumbbell "Skull Crusher" on Swiss Ball

Hold a pair of dumbbells and lie on the ball so that your head and neck are supported. Elevate your hips slightly and keep your abs tight. Extend the dumbbells straight up with your palms facing each other. Tilt your arms toward your head slightly, about 2 inches from straight up. Feather your breathing as you bend your elbows and lower the weights through a count of 10 seconds. Hold at the MTP, about an inch above your forehead, for 2 seconds. Raise dumbbells to starting point through a count of 10 seconds. Without resting, repeat three times.

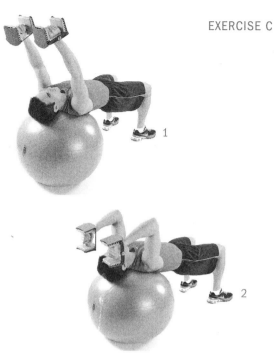

ABS

EXERCISE D

Swiss Ball Crunch

Sit on the ball with your feet on the floor. Walk your feet out until your hips are slightly lower than your knees but your lower back is still firmly supported. Place your hands behind your head to support your neck. Feather your breathing and, using your abs only, slowly crunch up through a count of 10 seconds. Hold and squeeze at the MTP for 2 seconds. Lower yourself to starting point through a count of 10 seconds. Without resting, repeat three times.

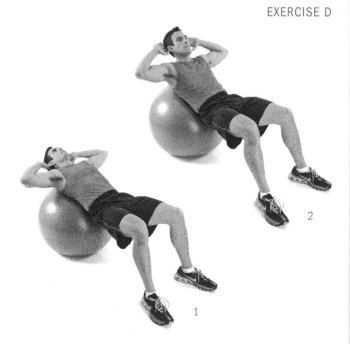

SHOULDERS

Seated Rear Delt Raise

Hold a pair of dumbbells and sit on the edge of a chair or bench. Lean forward until your chest is almost touching your knees and drop the dumbbells so your arms hang behind your heels, palms facing each other. Feather your breathing as you raise the weights up through a count of 10 seconds. Hold and squeeze for 2 seconds at the MTP. Return dumbbells to starting point through a count of 10 seconds. Without resting, repeat three times.

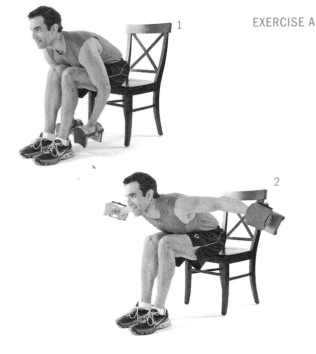

BICEPS

Preacher Curl on Swiss Ball

Hold a pair of dumbbells and rest over the ball with your knees on the floor and a 6- to 8-inch gap between your arms. Lift your arms to starting point with your elbows bent at about a 90-degree angle. Feather your breathing as you lower the weights through a count of 10 seconds. Hold at the MTP for a count of 2 seconds. Lift dumbbells to starting point through a count of 10 seconds. Without resting, repeat three times.

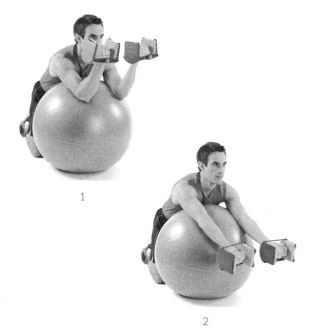

KEY: MTP: maximum tension point. **Feather your breathing:** Inhale deeply and exhale in short bursts.
Timing: Each exercise should take 90 seconds, and each circuit should take 6 minutes.

TRICEPS

EXERCISE C

Standing Triceps Kickback

Stand with a dumbbell in each hand, feet shoulder-width apart, and slightly bend your knees. Bend at the waist as if you were tying your shoe, and lift your head and chest, creating a slight arch in the back. Bend your arms and raise your elbows up as high as possible. Feather your breathing as you extend the dumbbells behind you through a count of 10 seconds. Hold and squeeze at the MTP for 2 seconds. Return to starting point through a count of 10 seconds. Without resting, repeat three times.

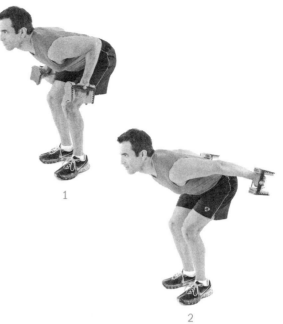

1

2

ABS

EXERCISE D

Lying Oblique Twist

Lie on your back with your arms outstretched, palms facing down. Raise your knees up to a 90-degree angle, and drop your knees down to one side. Feather your breathing as you rotate your knees to the other side through a count of 10 seconds. Hold and squeeze for 2 seconds at the MTP, about one inch from the ground. Then rotate to the other side through a count of 10 seconds. Without resting, repeat three times.

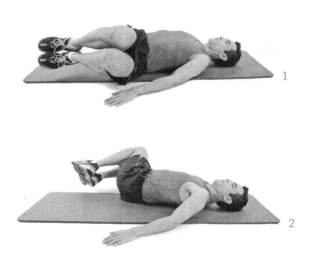

1

2

FINISH

LEGS

Chair Squat

Stand in front of a chair with your feet hip-width apart. Cross your arms, keeping your back straight, abs tight, and head up. Feather your breathing as you squat down as if you were about to sit in the chair through a count of 10 seconds. Hold for 2 seconds at the MTP, about 2 inches from touching the chair. Then push through your heels as you stand and return to starting point through a count of 10 seconds. Without resting, repeat three times.

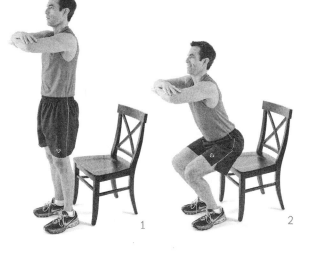

BACK

Pullover on Swiss Ball

Grasp a dumbbell using the diamond grip. Lie on the ball with your head and neck supported. Keep your hips up and abs tight throughout the exercise. Extend the weight over your chest with elbows slightly bent. Feather your breathing as you lower the weight down behind your head through a count of 10 seconds. Hold for 2 seconds at the MTP. Raise the dumbbell back to starting point through a count of 10 seconds. Without resting, repeat three times. (Note: How far you can stretch your arms back will determine your MTP.)

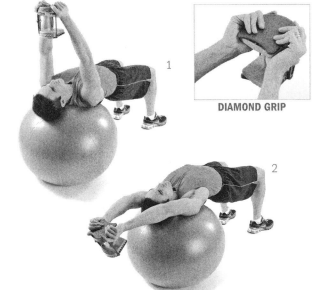

DIAMOND GRIP

KEY: MTP: maximum tension point. **Feather your breathing:** Inhale deeply and exhale in short bursts.
Timing: Each exercise should take 90 seconds, and each circuit should take 6 minutes.

CHEST

EXERCISE C

Incline Push-up

Lean against a wall or a set of stairs, so that your upper body is elevated above your feet. Keep your head up, back straight, and abs tight. Feather your breathing as you lower yourself down through a count of 10 seconds. Hold at the MTP for a count of 2 seconds. Return to starting point through a count of 10 seconds. Without resting, repeat three times.

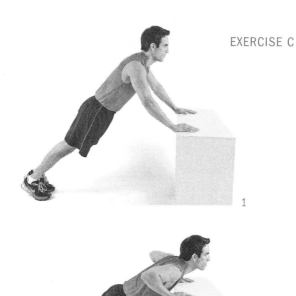

ABS

EXERCISE D

Reverse Crunch

Lie flat on a mat, with your hands by your sides, palms down. Pull your heels as close to your butt as possible. Raise your heels about 2 inches off the ground. Keep your chin up and abs tight. Feather your breathing as you pull your knees up using the lower abdominals through a count of 10 seconds. Hold and squeeze for 2 seconds at the MTP (when your butt is just off the ground). Lower your body to starting point through a 10-second count. Without resting, repeat three times.

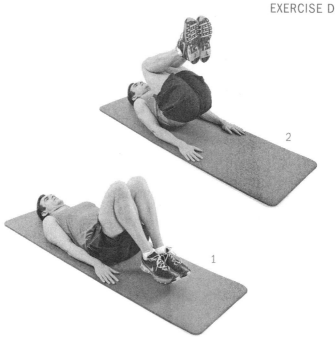

LEGS

Swiss Ball Squat

Place the ball against a sturdy wall and position yourself with the ball supporting your lower back. Stand with your feet hip-width apart, about 1 foot from the wall. Cross your arms in front of your shoulders. Feather your breathing as you squat through a count of 10 seconds to about a 90-degree angle. Hold at the MTP for a count of 2 seconds. Then drive through your heels, returning to starting point through a count of 10 seconds. Without resting, repeat three times.

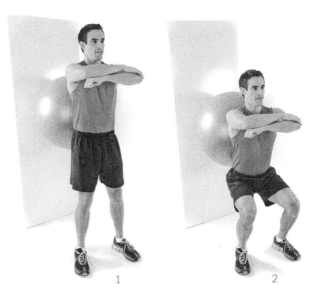

BACK

Bent-over Row (underhand grip)

Hold a pair of dumbbells, arms extended, using the underhand grip. Bend at the waist as if tying your shoes. Raise your head and chest to create a slight arch in the back. Bend your knees slightly. Feather your breathing as you pull the dumbbells up in a fluid rowing motion through a count of 10 seconds, keeping your elbows close to your body. Hold and squeeze your shoulder blades together at the MTP for 2 seconds. Lower your arms back to starting point through a count of 10. Without resting, repeat three times.

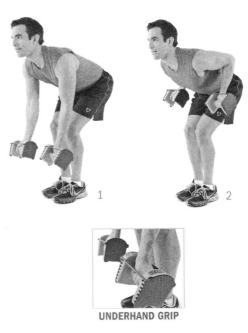

UNDERHAND GRIP

KEY: MTP: maximum tension point. **Feather your breathing:** Inhale deeply and exhale in short bursts.
Timing: Each exercise should take 90 seconds, and each circuit should take 6 minutes.

CHEST

Incline Dumbbell Fly on Swiss Ball

Hold a pair of dumbbells and lie on the ball with your head and neck supported. Roll down the ball until your hips drop almost to the ground. Extend the dumbbells over your chest, palms facing each other, elbows slightly bent. Feather your breathing as you lower the weights down and out through a count of 10 seconds. Hold for 2 seconds at the MTP. Raise the weight back to starting point in a "bear hug" motion through a count of 10 seconds. Without resting, repeat three times.

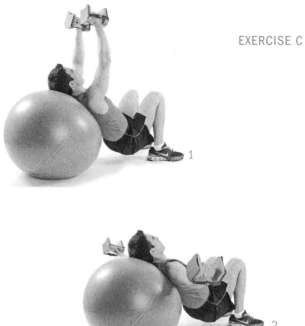

ABS

Swiss Ball Crunch with Elevated Feet

Sit on the ball about 2 feet away from a wall, hands behind your head. Walk your feet out, and place them against the wall. Feather your breathing as you crunch up through a count of 10 seconds, using only your abs. Hold and squeeze for 2 seconds at the MTP. Then return to starting point through a count of 10 seconds. Without resting, repeat three times. (Keep in mind that the range of motion is significantly shorter on this exercise, so be sure to adjust your pace.)

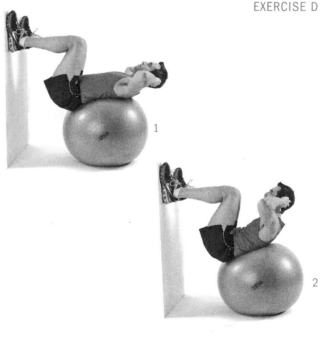

LEGS

EXERCISE A

Glute Kickback on Swiss Ball

Lie over the ball on your hands and knees. Press the heel of your foot toward the ceiling, keeping a bend in the knee, through a count of 10 seconds. Hold and squeeze for 2 seconds at the MTP. Then lower your leg back to starting point through a count of 10 seconds. Repeat once more on this leg. Without resting, switch sides and complete 2 more reps on the other side.

BACK

EXERCISE B

Reverse Hyperextension

Lie facedown on the ball. Roll yourself forward until the ball is under your hips and your upper body is angled toward the ground. Place your palms on the floor about shoulder-width apart. With legs together, feather your breathing as you raise your heels toward the ceiling, using your lower back and hamstrings. Raise through a count of 10 seconds. Hold and squeeze at the MTP for 2 seconds. With straight legs, lower through a count of 10 seconds to starting point, about 2 inches from the ground. Without resting, repeat three times.

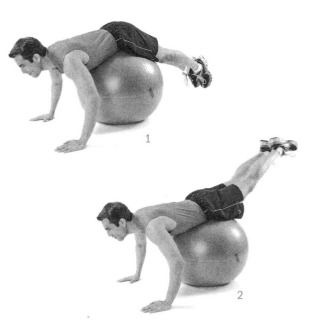

KEY: MTP: maximum tension point. **Feather your breathing:** Inhale deeply and exhale in short bursts.
Timing: Each exercise should take 90 seconds, and each circuit should take 6 minutes.

CHEST

EXERCISE C

Flat Press on Swiss Ball

Hold a pair of dumbbells and lie on the ball so that it comfortably supports your shoulder blades. Extend your arms in front of you, pressing the weights together. Feather your breathing as you lower the weights down through a count of 10 seconds. Hold for 2 seconds at MTP, about 1 inch above your chest. Press the dumbbells up and together back to starting point through a count of 10 seconds. Without resting, repeat three times.

ABS

EXERCISE D

Weighted Oblique Twist on Swiss Ball

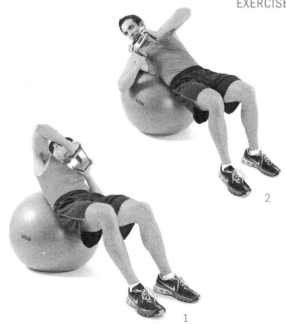

Sit on the ball, holding a dumbbell just under your chin. Walk your feet forward until your hips are slightly lower than your chest. Keep your abs tight and chin up. Turn to one side to begin the exercise. Slowly twist your torso to the other side through a count of 10. Hold and squeeze for 2 seconds at the MTP. Then twist to the other side through a count of 10 seconds. Without resting, repeat three times.

FINISH

SHOULDERS

EXERCISE A

Shoulder Press on Swiss Ball

Hold a pair of dumbbells and sit on the ball with your back straight, abs tight, and chin up. Extend the dumbbells up and together directly over your head, palms facing forward. Feather your breathing as you lower the weights down through a count of 10 seconds. Hold for 2 seconds at the MTP (chin level). Press the dumbbells up to starting point through a count of 10 seconds. Without resting, repeat three times.

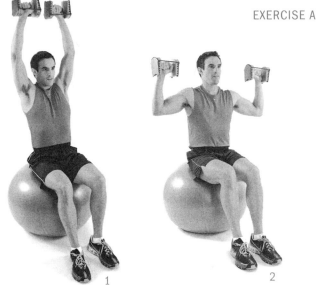

1   2

BICEPS

EXERCISE B

Side Curl on Swiss Ball

Hold a pair of dumbbells and sit on ball. With your arms out to your sides, palms turned up, and elbows tight against your body, feather your breathing as you curl the weights up through a count of 10 seconds. Hold and squeeze for a count of 2 seconds at the MTP. Lower the weight down to starting point through a count of 10 seconds. Without resting, repeat three times.

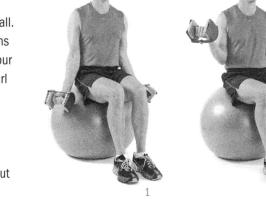

1   2

KEY: MTP: maximum tension point. **Feather your breathing:** Inhale deeply and exhale in short bursts.
Timing: Each exercise should take 90 seconds, and each circuit should take 6 minutes.

TRICEPS

EXERCISE C

Overhead Triceps Extension on Swiss Ball

Grasp a dumbbell using the diamond grip. Sit on the ball with your chest up, back straight, feet shoulder-width apart. Extend your arms, with your elbows slightly bent, keeping your biceps tight against your head. Feather your breathing as you lower the dumbbell through a count of 10 seconds. Hold for 2 seconds at the MTP when your elbows are at about a 90-degree angle. Press the weight up to return to starting point through a count of 10 seconds. Without resting, repeat three times.

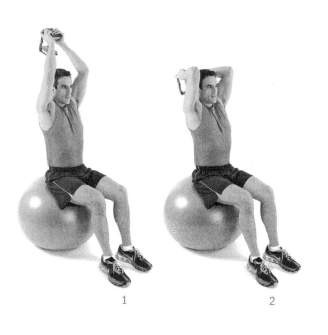

1   2

ABS

EXERCISE D

Toe Reach

Lie on your back. Cross your legs, flex your feet, and raise your legs to a 90-degree angle. Extend your arms and keep your chin up. Feather your breathing as you crunch up, reaching toward your toes through a count of 10 seconds. Hold for 2 seconds at the MTP, then lower yourself back to starting point through a count of 10 seconds. Keep your upper back from touching the ground. Without resting, repeat three times.

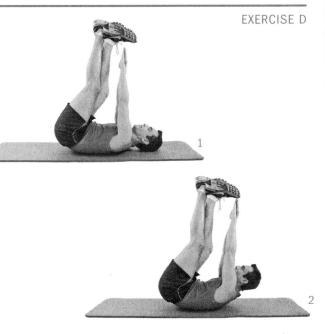

SHOULDERS

EXERCISE A

Seated Rear Delt Raise

Hold a pair of dumbbells and sit on the edge of a chair or a bench. Lean forward until your chest is almost touching your knees, and let the dumbbells hang just behind your heels, your palms facing each other. Feather your breathing as you raise the weights up through a count of 10 seconds. Hold and squeeze for 2 seconds at the MTP. Return dumbbells to starting point through a count of 10 seconds. Without resting, repeat three times.

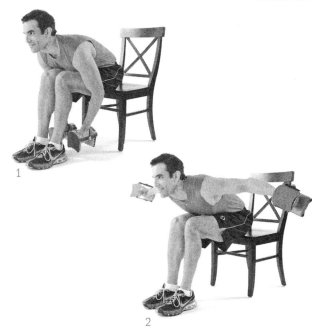

BICEPS

EXERCISE B

Preacher Curl on Swiss Ball

Hold a pair of dumbbells and rest over the ball with your knees on the floor and a 6- to 8-inch gap between your arms. Lift your arms to starting point with your elbows bent at about a 90-degree angle. Feather your breathing as you lower the weights through a count of 10 seconds. Hold at the MTP for a count of 2 seconds. Lift dumbbells to starting point through a count of 10 seconds. Without resting, repeat three times.

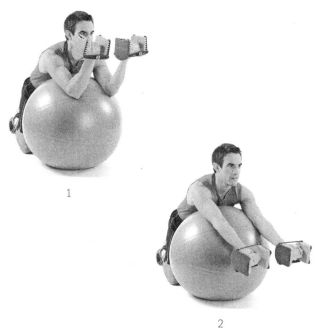

KEY: MTP: maximum tension point. **Feather your breathing:** Inhale deeply and exhale in short bursts.
Timing: Each exercise should take 90 seconds, and each circuit should take 6 minutes.

TRICEPS

Close-Grip Diamond Push-up on Knees

Lie flat on a mat or towel using the diamond position. Cross your ankles as you balance on your knees and extend your arms. Keeping your back straight and abs tight, feather your breathing as you lower your body through a count of 10 seconds, allowing your elbows to move outward. Hold for 2 seconds at the MTP, about 2 inches above the ground. Return to starting position through a count of 10 seconds. Without resting, repeat three times.

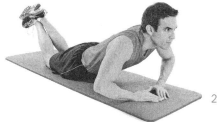
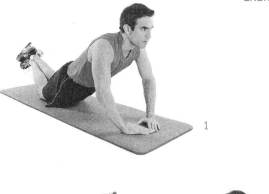

ABS

Seated V-up

Sit on the ground with your arms slightly behind you, elbows bent, and fingertips pointed toward your body. Start with your knees together, legs extended, and heels off the ground about 2 inches. Lean your upper body weight back on your palms just slightly. Feather your breathing as you pull your knees into your chest for a count of 10. Hold and squeeze 2 seconds at the MTP. Return to starting point through a count of 10, keeping your abs tight. Without resting, repeat three times.

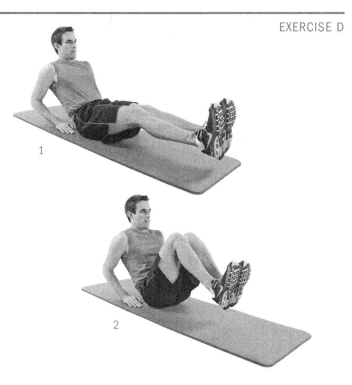

SHOULDERS

Reverse Lateral

Hold a pair of dumbbells and sit on the ball with your back straight and your abs tight. Extend your arms over your head with a slight bend in the elbows, palms facing each other. Feather your breathing as you lower the weights down and out to your sides for a count of 10, keeping the palms up the entire movement. Hold for 2 seconds at the MTP, where your arms are parallel to the ground. Return to starting point through a count of 10 seconds. Without resting, repeat three times.

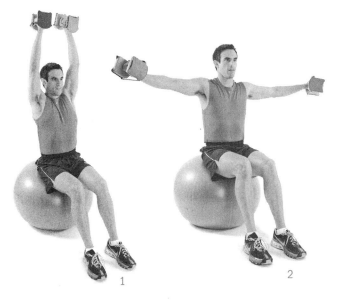

BICEPS

Standing Hammer Curl

Hold a pair of dumbbells and stand with your feet shoulder-width apart and your arms extended by your sides, palms facing each other, knees slightly bent. Feather your breathing as you curl the weights up through a count of 10 seconds, keeping your palms facing each other. Hold and squeeze at the MTP for 2 seconds. Lower the weight to starting point through a count of 10 seconds. Without resting, repeat three times.

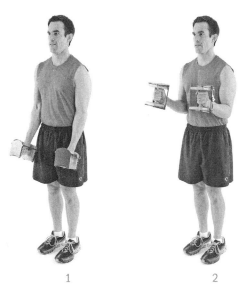

KEY: **MTP:** maximum tension point. **Feather your breathing:** Inhale deeply and exhale in short bursts.
Timing: Each exercise should take 90 seconds, and each circuit should take 6 minutes.

TRICEPS

Chair Dip

Sit on the front edge of a sturdy chair or bench, hands close by your sides and fingers forward. With your legs extended, flex your feet so that your weight is on your heels. Feather your breathing as you slide away from the chair and lower yourself down for a count of 10 seconds. Hold for 2 seconds at the MTP. (Note: This point will depend on how flexible your shoulders are. Your MTP will be about an inch above your most flexible point.) Lift yourself back up to starting point through a count 10 seconds. Without resting, repeat three times.

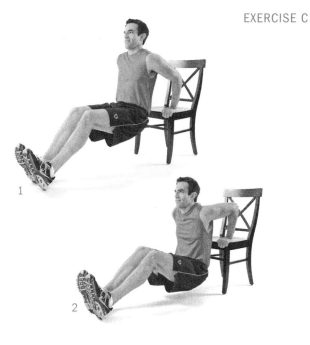

ABS

Russian Twist

Sit on the floor or on a mat with your knees bent, feet together. Keep your chin up and abs tight as you lean back slightly, engaging your abs. Extend your arms out away from your chest with your palms pressed together and turned to one side to begin the exercise. Feather your breathing as you slowly rotate your torso as far as possible to the other side through a count of 10 seconds. Hold and squeeze at the MTP for 2 seconds. Rotate back to the other side through a count of 10 seconds. Without resting, repeat three times.

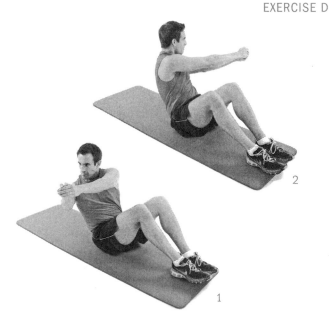

FINISH

ADVANCED PHASE

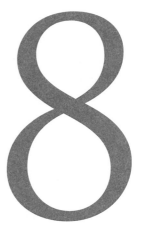

WEEKS 3 TO 8

START

LEGS

EXERCISE A

Plié Squat

Hold one dumbbell with both hands and stand with your feet about twice shoulder-width apart, toes turned out to the sides and knees aligned over the toes. Feather your breathing as you squat through a count of 10 seconds. Hold for 2 seconds at the MTP. Push through your heels to return to starting point through a count of 10 seconds. Without resting, repeat three times.

1

2

BACK

EXERCISE B

Pullover on Swiss Ball

Grasp a dumbbell using the diamond grip. Lie on the ball with your head and neck supported. Keep your hips up and abs tight throughout the exercise. Extend the weight over your chest with a slight bend in the elbows. Feather your breathing as you lower the weight down behind your head through a count of 10 seconds. Hold for 2 seconds at the MTP. Raise the weight back to starting point through a count of 10 seconds. Without resting, repeat three times. (Note: How far you can stretch your arms back will determine your MTP.)

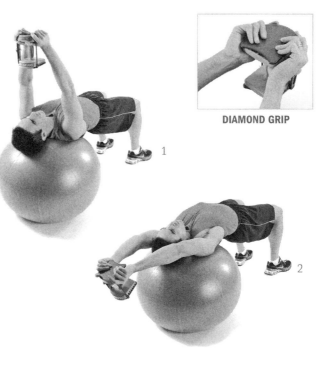

DIAMOND GRIP

1

2

KEY: MTP: maximum tension point. **Feather your breathing:** Inhale deeply and exhale in short bursts.
Timing: Each exercise should take 90 seconds, and each circuit should take 6 minutes.

CHEST

EXERCISE C

Flat Dumbbell Fly on Swiss Ball

Hold a pair of dumbbells and lie on the ball with your head and neck supported. Extend the dumbbells over your chest, palms facing each other, elbows slightly bent. Feather your breathing as you lower the weights down and out through a count of 10 seconds. Hold for two seconds at the MTP. Raise the weight back to starting point in a "bear hug" motion through a count of 10 seconds. Without resting, repeat three times.

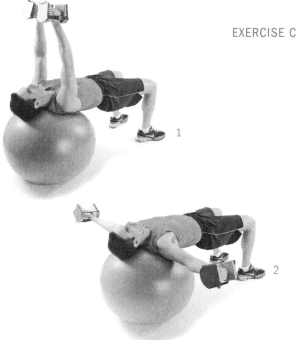

ABS

EXERCISE D

Chair Crunch

Sit on a chair or exercise bench. Reach your hands behind you and grab the sides of the chair. Extend your legs out and allow your upper body to recline back slightly. Feather your breathing as you draw your knees in and up toward your chin through a 10-second count. Hold and squeeze for 2 seconds at the MTP. Return to starting point through a count of 10 seconds. Without resting, repeat three times.

LEGS

EXERCISE A

Quadriceps Flex

Stand with feet shoulder-width apart. Grasp a chair or support at about hip level. Feather your breathing as you bend your knees and allow your body to fall backward, letting your heels come off the floor, through a count of 10 seconds. Hold and squeeze your quads for 2 seconds at the MTP (when your knees are near the floor). Return to starting point through a count of 10 seconds. Without resting, repeat three times.

BACK

EXERCISE B

Bent-over Row (standard grip)

Hold a pair of dumbbells, arms extended, palms facing each other. Bend at the waist as if tying your shoes. Raise your head and chest to create a slight arch in the back. Bend your knees slightly. Feather your breathing as you pull the dumbbells up in a fluid rowing motion through a count of 10 seconds, keeping your elbows close to your body. Hold and squeeze your shoulder blades together at the MTP for 2 seconds. Lower your arms back to starting point through a count of 10 seconds. Without resting, repeat three times.

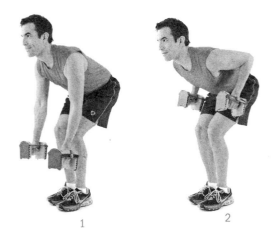

KEY: **MTP:** maximum tension point. **Feather your breathing:** Inhale deeply and exhale in short bursts.
Timing: Each exercise should take 90 seconds, and each circuit should take 6 minutes.

CHEST

Incline Push-up

Lean against a wall or a set of stairs, so that your upper body is elevated above your feet. Keep your head up, back straight, and abs tight. Feather your breathing as you lower yourself down through a count of 10. Hold at the MTP for 2 seconds. Return to starting point through a count of 10 seconds. Without resting, repeat three times.

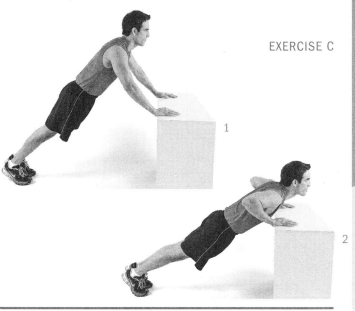

ABS

Double Crunch

Lie on a mat or towel. Place your hands behind your head. Pull your heels toward your butt as far as you can. Keep your elbows and chin up, abs tight. Using your upper abs, feather your breathing as you crunch up while simultaneously pulling your knees in through a count of 10 seconds. Hold and squeeze at the MTP for 2 seconds. Return to starting point through a count of 10 seconds, never letting your upper back touch the ground. Without resting, repeat three times. (Note: The range of motion on this exercise is very short, so be sure to adjust your speed so that you hit the MTP on the count of 10.)

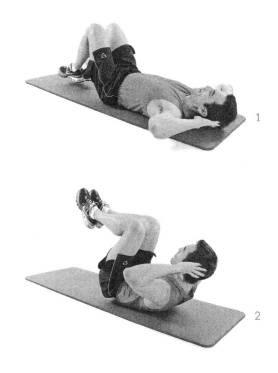

LEGS

EXERCISE A

Lunge

Stand in a lunge position. Keep your back straight, chest up, and abs tight. Feather your breathing as you drop your back knee toward the ground through a count of 10 seconds. Hold for 2 seconds at the MTP, about 1 inch above the ground. Return to starting position through a count of 10 seconds. Without resting, repeat one more time on this leg, then perform 2 more reps on the other leg, for a total of 4 reps. (Note: To avoid injury, make sure that your front knee stays aligned with your toes and doesn't bend farther than a 90-degree angle.)

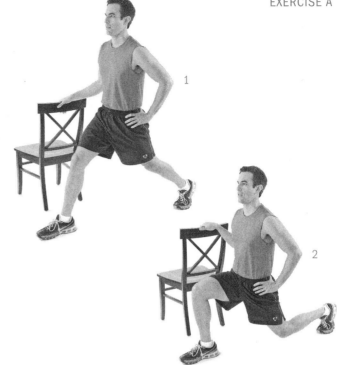

BACK

EXERCISE B

Hyperextension on Swiss Ball

Lie on the ball, bending at the waist, with your hips supported and your hands behind your head. Feather your breathing as you lift your upper body through a count of 10 seconds, using your lower back muscles to perform the movement. Hold for 2 seconds at the MTP. Return to starting point through a count of 10 seconds. Without resting, repeat three times.

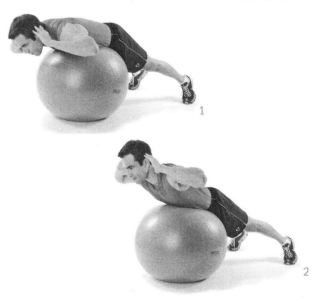

KEY: MTP: maximum tension point. **Feather your breathing:** Inhale deeply and exhale in short bursts.
Timing: Each exercise should take 90 seconds, and each circuit should take 6 minutes.

CHEST

Incline Press on Swiss Ball

Hold a pair of dumbbells and lie on the ball so that your head and neck are supported. Allow your hips to drop almost to the ground. Press the weights up and together, with a slight bend in the elbows, so that the upper chest is targeted. Feather your breathing as you lower the weights through a count of 10 seconds. Hold for 2 seconds at the MTP. Press the dumbbells up to starting point through a count of 10 seconds. Without resting, repeat three times.

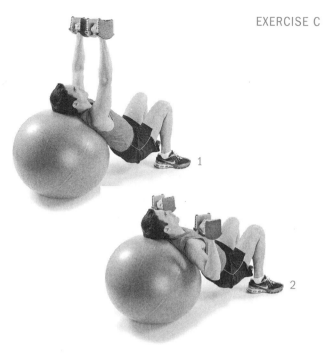

ABS

Weighted Oblique Twist on Swiss Ball

Hold a dumbbell just under your chin and sit on the ball. Walk your feet forward until your hips are slightly lower than your chest. Keep your abs tight and chin up. Turn to one side to begin the exercise. Slowly twist your torso to the other side through a count of 10 seconds. Hold and squeeze for 2 seconds at the MTP. Then twist to the other side through a count of 10 seconds. Without resting, repeat three times.

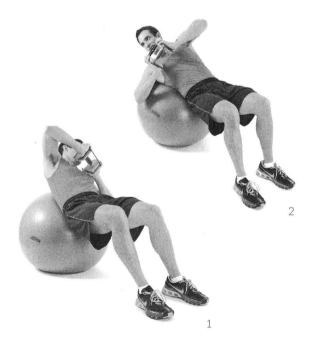

FINISH

SHOULDERS

EXERCISE A

Standing Shoulder Press

Hold a pair of dumbbells and stand with your back straight, abs tight, and chin up. Extend the weights up and together directly over your head, palms facing forward. Feather your breathing as you lower the weights down through a count of 10 seconds. Hold for 2 seconds at the MTP (chin level). Press the dumbbells up to starting point through a count of 10 seconds. Without resting, repeat three times.

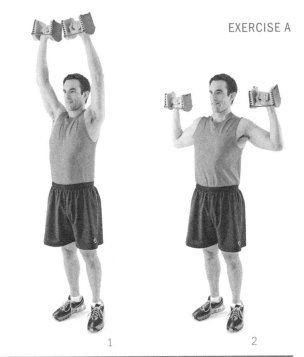

1

2

BICEPS

EXERCISE B

Standing Side Curl

Hold a pair of dumbbells with your palms turned out, elbows to your sides. Keep your chest up, feet hip-width apart, knees slightly bent, and abs tight throughout the exercise. Feather your breathing as you curl the weights up through a count of 10 seconds. Hold and squeeze at the MTP for a count of 2 seconds, then lower the weights down to starting point through a count of 10 seconds, until your arms are completely straight (do not lock your elbows). Without resting, repeat three times. (Note: As you perform the exercise, be sure to keep your elbows tight against your body.)

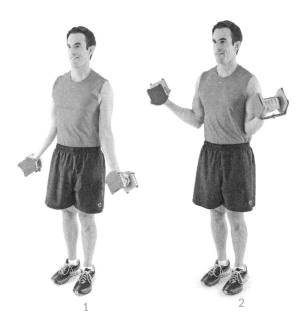

1

2

KEY: MTP: maximum tension point. **Feather your breathing:** Inhale deeply and exhale in short bursts.
Timing: Each exercise should take 90 seconds, and each circuit should take 6 minutes.

TRICEPS

EXERCISE C

"Skull Crusher" on Swiss Ball

Hold a pair of dumbbells and lie on the ball so that your head and neck are supported. Keep your hips up and abs tight throughout the exercise. Extend the dumbbells over your head with elbows slightly bent, palms facing each other. Drop your arms back slightly, about 2 inches. Feather your breathing as you bend your elbows and lower the weights down through a count of 10 seconds. Hold at the MTP for 2 seconds, about an inch above your forehead. Raise the weight back to starting point through a count of 10. Without resting, repeat three times.

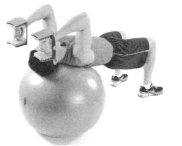

ABS

EXERCISE D

Crunch with Feet Elevated on Swiss Ball

Lie on the ground with your feet on the ball, knees bent. Keep your back straight, abs tight, and place your hands behind your head to support your neck. Keep your chin up and feather your breathing as you crunch up toward your knees for a count of 10 seconds. Hold and squeeze at the MTP for 2 seconds. Return to starting point through a count of 10 seconds. Without resting, repeat three times.

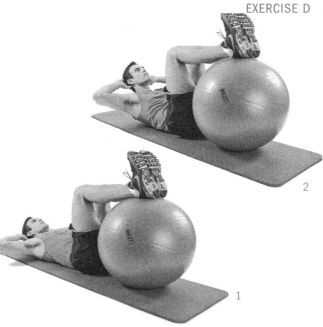

SHOULDERS

Front Delt Raise on Swiss Ball

Hold a pair of dumbbells and stand with a ball against a sturdy wall, the ball between your shoulder blades, and your body slightly angled back toward the wall. Feather your breathing as you raise the dumbbells with slightly bent elbows for a count of 10 seconds. Hold for 2 seconds at the MTP (about eye level). Lower the weights back to starting point through a count of 10 seconds. Without resting, repeat three times.

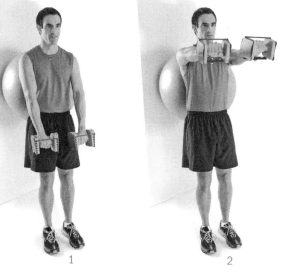

1

2

BICEPS

Standing Biceps Curl on Swiss Ball

Hold a pair of dumbbells and stand with a ball against a sturdy wall, the ball between your shoulder blades and the top of your hips. Bend your knees slightly. Keep your abs tight and chest up. Feather your breathing as you curl the weights up through a count of 10 seconds. Hold and squeeze for 2 seconds at the MTP. Lower the weights back to starting point through a count of 10 seconds, until your arms are completely straight at the bottom. Without resting, repeat three times. (Note: As you perform the exercises, be sure not to let your elbows move away from your body.)

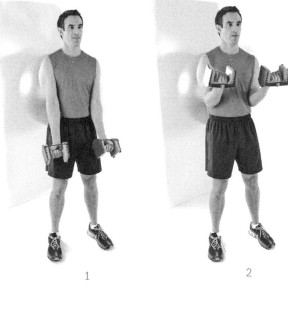

1

2

KEY: MTP: maximum tension point. **Feather your breathing:** Inhale deeply and exhale in short bursts.
Timing: Each exercise should take 90 seconds, and each circuit should take 6 minutes.

TRICEPS

EXERCISE C

Chair Dip with Swiss Ball

Sit on the front edge of a sturdy chair or exercise bench, hands close by your sides, fingers forward, and legs extended resting on the ball. Feather your breathing as you lower yourself down through a count of 10 seconds. Hold at the MTP for 2 seconds. Push yourself back up to starting point through a count of 10 seconds. Without resting, repeat three times. (Note: The MTP will depend on how flexible your shoulders are. Your MTP will be about an inch above your most flexible point. Also, if this exercise is too difficult, use the previous version of this exercise without the ball on page 85.)

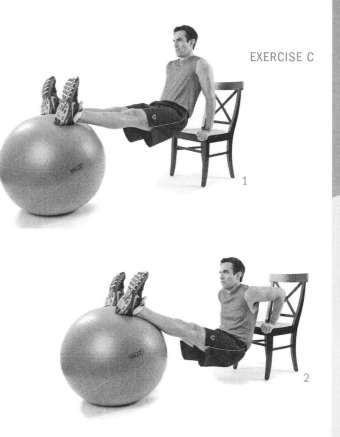

ABS

EXERCISE D

Reverse Crunch

Lie flat on the floor with your hands down by your sides, palms down. Keep your chin tucked in and abs tight. Feather your breathing as you pull your knees up slowly toward your chin through a count of 10 seconds. Hold for 2 seconds at the MTP (when the hips are off the ground slightly). Lower your body to starting point through a count of 10 seconds. Without resting, repeat three times.

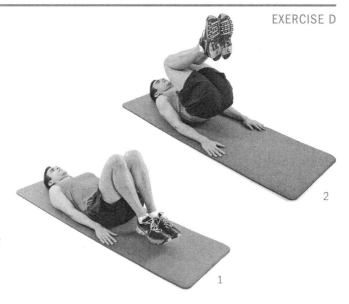

SHOULDERS

EXERCISE A

Bent-over Rear Delt Raise

Hold a pair of dumbbells, palms facing each other. Bend at the waist as if you were about to tie your shoes, then lift only your chin and chest, creating a slight arch in your back. Feather your breathing as you raise the weights up to the sides through a count of 10 seconds. Hold and squeeze for 2 seconds at the MTP. Lower the weights to starting point through a count of 10 seconds. Without resting, repeat three times.

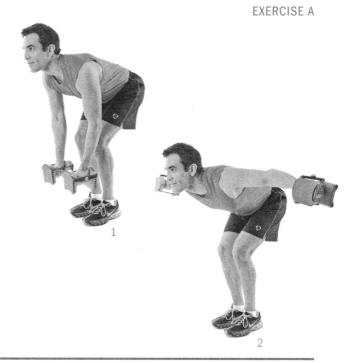

BICEPS

EXERCISE B

Standing Hammer Curl

Hold a pair of dumbbells and stand with your feet shoulder-width apart, knees slightly bent, and arms extended downward by your sides, palms facing in toward your body. Feather your breathing as you curl the weights up through a count of 10 seconds, keeping your palms facing each other. Hold and squeeze at the MTP for 2 seconds. Lower the weights to starting point through a count of 10 seconds. Without resting, repeat three times.

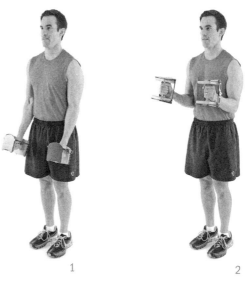

KEY: **MTP:** maximum tension point. **Feather your breathing:** Inhale deeply and exhale in short bursts. **Timing:** Each exercise should take 90 seconds, and each circuit should take 6 minutes.

TRICEPS

EXERCISE C

Standing Triceps Kickback

Hold a pair of dumbbells, palms facing each other. Bend at the waist as if you were about to tie your shoes, then lift only your chin and chest, creating a slight arch in your back, and slightly bend your knees. Raise your elbows as high as possible, while keeping them close to your body. Feather your breathing as you extend the weights back and out (without moving the upper part of the arm) through a count of 10 seconds. Hold and squeeze at the MTP for 2 seconds. Return the weights to starting point through a count of 10 seconds. Without resting, repeat three times.

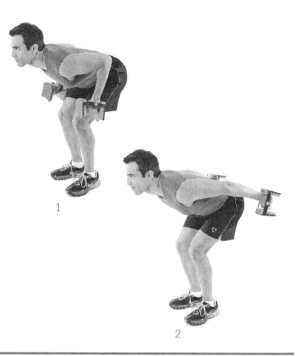

ABS

EXERCISE D

Bicycle Crunch

Lie flat on your back. Place your hands behind your head and raise your heels about 2 inches from the ground, keeping your chin up and abs tight throughout the exercise. Bring your right elbow to your left knee and feather your breathing as you rotate to the other side for a count of 10 seconds. Hold and squeeze for 2 seconds at the MTP (where your left elbow meets your right knee). Lower your body to starting point through a count of 10 seconds. Without resting, repeat three times, alternating sides, for a total of 2 reps per side.

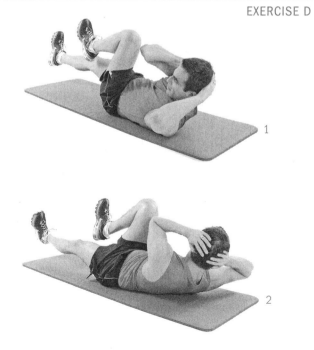

FINISH

LEGS

EXERCISE A

Lateral Squat

Take a stance about a foot wider than shoulder-width on each side. Feather your breathing as you squat down toward one leg, while keeping the opposite leg straight through a count of 10 seconds. Hold for 2 seconds at the MTP. Return to starting point through a count of 10 seconds. Without resting, alternate sides and complete 2 reps on each side for a total of 4.

1

2

BACK

EXERCISE B

Pullover on Swiss Ball

Grasp a dumbbell using the diamond grip. Lie on the ball with your head and neck supported. Keep your hips up and abs tight throughout the exercise. Extend the weight over your chest with a slight bend in the elbows. Feather your breathing as you lower the weight down behind your head through a count of 10 seconds. Hold for 2 seconds at the MTP. Raise the weight back to starting point through a count of 10 seconds. Without resting, repeat three times. (Note: How far you can stretch your arms back will determine your MTP.)

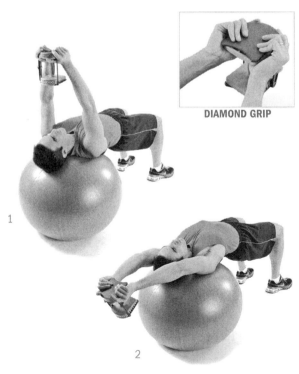

DIAMOND GRIP

1

2

KEY: MTP: maximum tension point. **Feather your breathing:** Inhale deeply and exhale in short bursts.
Timing: Each exercise should take 90 seconds, and each circuit should take 6 minutes.

CHEST

EXERCISE C

Incline Push-up

Lean against a wall or a set of stairs, so that your upper body is elevated above your feet. Keep your head up, back straight, and abs tight. Feather your breathing as you lower yourself through a count of 10 seconds. Hold at the MTP for 2 seconds. Return to starting point through a count of 10 seconds. Without resting, repeat three times.

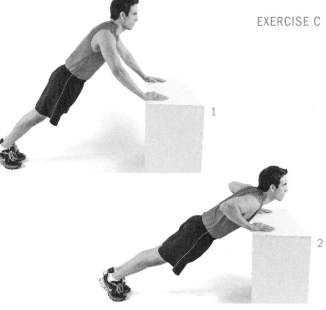

ABS

EXERCISE D

Double Crunch

Lie on a mat or towel. Place your hands behind your head, elbows and chin up, and abs tight. Pull your heels toward your butt as far as you can. Using your upper abs, feather your breathing as you crunch up while simultaneously pulling your knees in through a count of 10 seconds. Hold and squeeze at the MTP for 2 seconds. Return to starting position through a count of 10 seconds, never letting your upper back touch the ground. Without resting, repeat three times. (Note: The range of motion on this exercise is very short so be sure to adjust your speed so that you hit the MTP on the count of 10.)

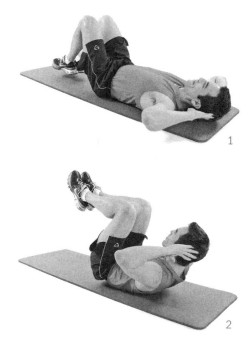

LEGS

Chair Squat

Stand in front of a chair with your feet hip-width apart. Cross your arms, keep your back straight, abs tight, and head up. Feather your breathing as you squat as if you were about to sit in the chair through a count of 10 seconds. Hold for 2 seconds at the MTP, about 2 inches from touching the chair. Then push through your heels as you stand and return to starting point through a count of 10 seconds. Without resting, repeat three times.

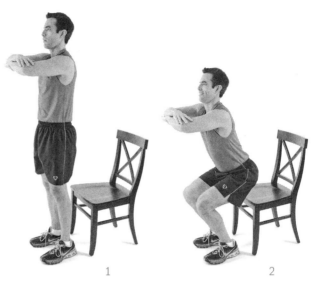

BACK

Swiss Ball Row

Hold a pair of dumbbells and lie on the ball so that it is at the middle of your waist. Raise your head and chest, creating a slight arch in the back. Feather your breathing as you pull the dumbbells up and back toward your hips in a rowing motion through a count of 10 seconds. Hold and squeeze your shoulder blades together at the MTP for 2 seconds. Return to starting point through a count of 10 seconds. Without resting, repeat three times.

KEY: **MTP:** maximum tension point. **Feather your breathing:** Inhale deeply and exhale in short bursts.
Timing: Each exercise should take 90 seconds, and each circuit should take 6 minutes.

CHEST EXERCISE C

Flat Press on Swiss Ball

Hold a pair of dumbbells and lie on the ball so that it comfortably supports your shoulder blades. Extend your arms in front of you, pressing the weights together. Feather your breathing as you lower the weights through a count of 10 seconds. Hold for 2 seconds at MTP, about 1 inch above your chest. Press the dumbbells up and together back to starting point through a count of 10 seconds. Without resting, repeat three times.

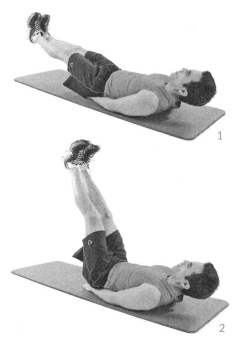

ABS EXERCISE D

Leg Lift

Lie on your back with your palms down, hands underneath your butt. Crunch up and hold your upper abs tight so that your shoulder blades are off the ground. Lift your legs about 2 inches off the ground. Keep your abs tight and chin up, and feather your breathing as you lift your legs through a count of 10 seconds. Hold and squeeze at the MTP for 2 seconds. Lower your legs to starting point through a count of 10 seconds. Without resting, repeat three times.

LEGS

Lunge

Stand with about a 2-foot gap between your front and back leg. Keep your back straight, chest up, and abs tight. Feather your breathing as you drop your back knee toward the ground through a count of 10 seconds. Hold for 2 seconds at the MTP, about 1 inch above the ground. Return back to starting position through a count of 10 seconds. Without resting, repeat one more time on this leg, then perform 2 more reps on the other side, for a total of 4 reps. (Note: To avoid injury, make sure that your front knee stays aligned with your toes and doesn't bend farther than a 90-degree angle.)

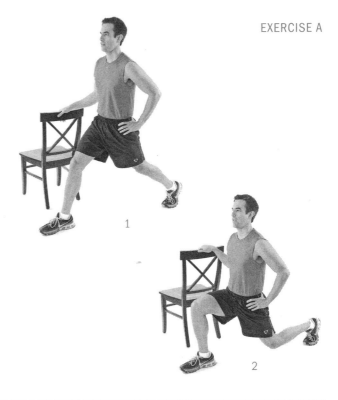

BACK

Reverse Hyperextension on Swiss Ball

Lie facedown on the ball. Roll yourself forward until the ball is under your hips and your upper body is angled toward the ground. Place your palms on the floor about shoulder-width apart. Keep your feet together and legs straight as you place your feet about 2 inches from the ground. Feather your breathing as you raise your heels toward the ceiling, using your lower back and hamstrings, through a count of 10 seconds. Hold and squeeze at the MTP for 2 seconds. Lower your heels back to starting point through a count of 10 seconds. Without resting, repeat three times.

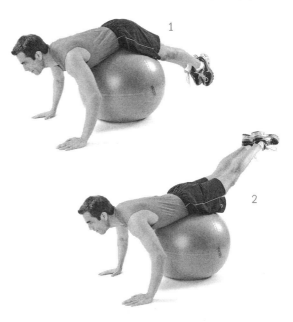

KEY: **MTP:** maximum tension point. **Feather your breathing:** Inhale deeply and exhale in short bursts.
Timing: Each exercise should take 90 seconds, and each circuit should take 6 minutes.

CHEST

Incline Dumbbell Fly on Swiss Ball

Hold a pair of dumbbells and lie on the ball with your head and neck supported. Roll down the ball until your hips drop almost to the ground. Extend the dumbbells over your chest, palms facing each other, elbows slightly bent. Feather your breathing as you lower the weights down and out through a count of 10 seconds. Hold for 2 seconds at the MTP. Raise the weights back to starting point in a "bear hug" motion through a count of 10 seconds. Without resting, repeat three times.

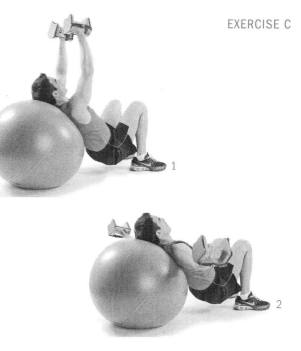

ABS

Russian Twist

Sit on the floor or mat with your knees bent, feet together. Keep your chin up and abs tight as you lean back slightly, engaging your abs. Extend your arms away from your chest with your palms pressed together and turn to one side to begin the exercise. Feather your breathing as you slowly rotate your torso as far as possible to the other side through a count of 10 seconds. Hold and squeeze at the MTP for 2 seconds. Rotate back to the other side through a count of 10 seconds. Without resting, repeat three times.

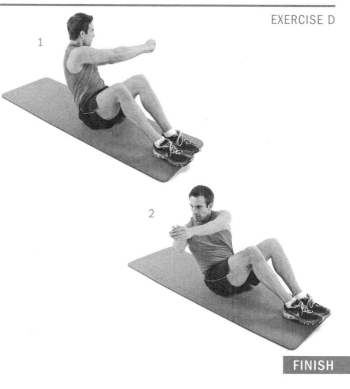

FINISH

SHOULDERS

Reverse Lateral on Swiss Ball

Hold a pair of dumbbells and sit on the ball with your back straight and your abs tight. Extend your arms over your head with a slight bend in the elbows, palms facing each other. Feather your breathing as you lower the weights down and out to your sides through a count of 10 seconds, keeping your palms up throughout the entire movement. Hold for 2 seconds at the MTP, when your arms are parallel to the ground. Then return to starting point through a count of 10 seconds. Without resting, repeat three times.

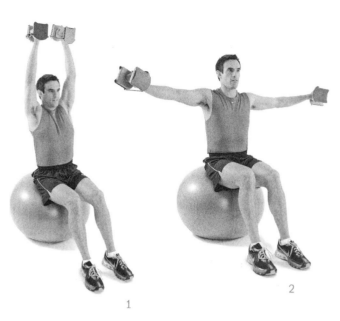

1

2

BICEPS

Standing Curl

Hold a pair of dumbbells, palms facing out. Stand with your feet shoulder-width apart and your arms extended by your sides, knees slightly bent. Feather your breathing as you curl the dumbbells up through a count of 10 seconds. Hold and squeeze for 2 seconds at the MTP. Keep your elbows tight against your body as you lower the weights for 10 seconds to starting point. Without resting, repeat three times. (Note: Be sure not to let your elbows move away from your sides through the entire exercise.)

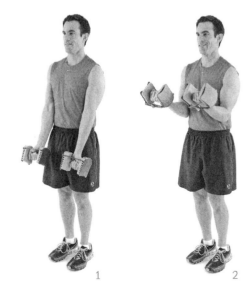

1

2

KEY: MTP: maximum tension point. **Feather your breathing:** Inhale deeply and exhale in short bursts.
Timing: Each exercise should take 90 seconds, and each circuit should take 6 minutes.

TRICEPS

Standing Triceps Kickback

Stand holding a pair of dumbbells, palms facing in, feet shoulder-width apart, and your knees slightly bent. Bend at the waist as if you were tying your shoes, and raise your head and chest, creating a slight arch in your back. With your elbows raised as high as possible, feather your breathing as you extend the dumbbells out through a count of 10 seconds. Hold and squeeze at the MTP for 2 seconds. Return to starting position through a count of 10 seconds. Without resting, repeat three times.

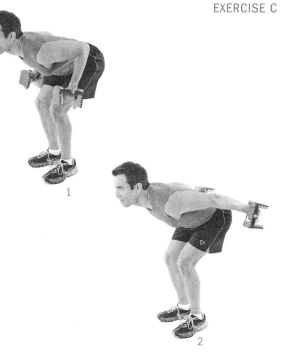

ABS

Swiss Ball Crunch with Elevated Feet

Sit on the ball about 2 feet away from a wall, arms crossed. Walk your feet out, and place them against the wall. Feather your breathing as you crunch up through a count of 10 seconds, using only your abs. Hold and squeeze for 2 seconds at the MTP. Then return to starting point through a count of 10 seconds. Without resting, repeat three times. (Note: Keep in mind that the range of motion is short on this exercise, so be sure to adjust your pace.)

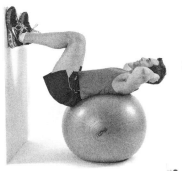

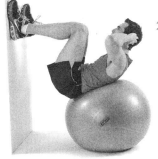

SHOULDERS

Upright Row

Hold a pair of dumbbells and stand with your feet together and slightly bent, and your arms extended down in front of you with a slight bend in your elbows, palms facing your body. Feather your breathing as you draw the weights up toward your chin through a count of 10 seconds. Hold for 2 seconds at the MTP, right below your chin. Return to starting point through a count of 10 seconds. Without resting, repeat three times. (Note: You should not feel a strain in your neck; if you do, relax your neck muscles and focus the exertion on your shoulders.)

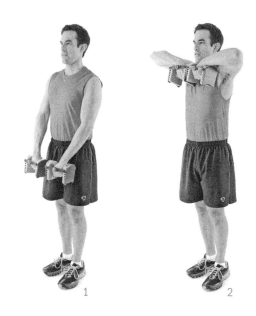

BICEPS

Standing Side Curl

Hold a pair of dumbbells with your palms turned out, your elbows tight against your body. Keep your chest up, feet hip-width apart, knees slightly bent, and abs tight throughout the exercise. Feather your breathing as you curl the weights up toward your shoulders for a count of 10 seconds, keeping your elbows tight against your body. Hold and squeeze at the MTP for a count of 2 seconds. Lower the weights through a count of 10 seconds until your arms are nearly straight (do not lock your elbows). Without resting, repeat three times.

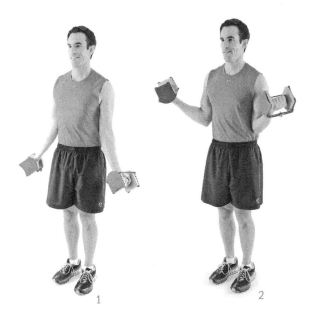

KEY: MTP: maximum tension point. **Feather your breathing:** Inhale deeply and exhale in short bursts.
Timing: Each exercise should take 90 seconds, and each circuit should take 6 minutes.

TRICEPS

EXERCISE C

Dumbbell "Skull Crusher" on Swiss Ball

Hold a pair of dumbbells and lie on the ball so that your head and neck are supported. Elevate your hips slightly and keep your abs tight. Extend the dumbbells straight up with your palms facing each other. Tilt your arms toward your head slightly, about 2 inches from straight up. Feather your breathing as you bend your elbows and lower the weights down through a count of 10 seconds. Hold at the MTP, about an inch above your forehead, for 2 seconds. Raise the dumbbells to starting point through a count of 10 seconds. Without resting, repeat three times.

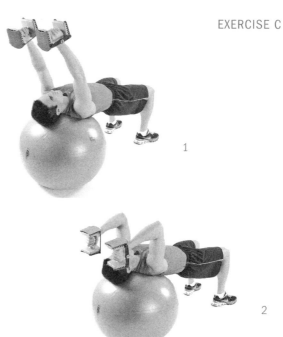

ABS

EXERCISE D

Seated V-up

Sit on the ground with your arms slightly behind you, elbows bent, and fingertips pointed toward your body. Start with your knees together, legs extended, and heels about 2 inches off the ground. Lean your upper body weight back on your palms just slightly. Feather your breathing as you pull your knees into your chest for a count of 10 seconds. Hold and squeeze 2 seconds at the MTP. Return to starting point through a count of 10 seconds, keeping your abs tight. Without resting, repeat three times.

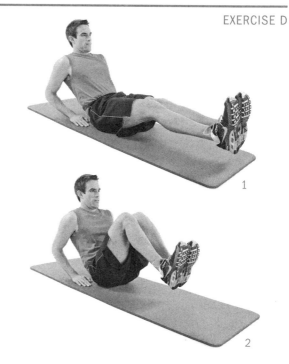

SHOULDERS

EXERCISE A

Chicken Wing

Hold a pair of dumbbells and stand hip-width apart and knees slightly bent. Bend your elbows (as pictured), holding the dumbbells in front of you at a 45-degree angle. Keep your forearms tight and feather your breathing as you raise your elbows out and up through a count of 10 seconds. Hold and squeeze for 2 seconds at the MTP. Return to starting point through a count of 10 seconds. Without resting, repeat three times. (Note: Be sure to relax your neck and avoid shrugging your shoulders.)

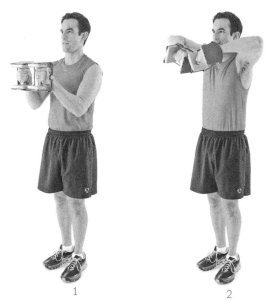

1   2

BICEPS

EXERCISE B

Preacher Curl on Swiss Ball

Hold a pair of dumbbells and rest over the ball with your knees on the floor and a 6- to 8-inch gap between your arms. Lift your arms to starting point, with your elbows bent at about a 90-degree angle. Feather your breathing as you lower the weights through a count of 10 seconds. Hold at the MTP for a count of 2 seconds. Lift dumbbells to starting point through a count of 10 seconds. Without resting, repeat three times.

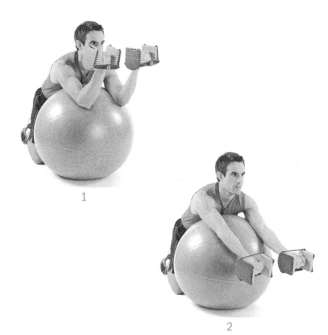

1   2

KEY: MTP: maximum tension point. **Feather your breathing:** Inhale deeply and exhale in short bursts.
Timing: Each exercise should take 90 seconds, and each circuit should take 6 minutes.

TRICEPS

EXERCISE C

Chair Dip with Swiss Ball

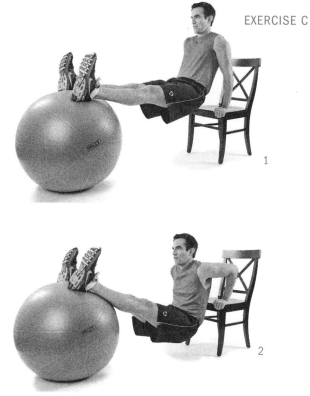

Sit on the front edge of a sturdy chair or exercise bench, hands close by your sides, fingers forward, and legs extended on a Swiss ball. Feather your breathing as you lower yourself through a count of 10 seconds. Hold at the MTP for 2 seconds. Push yourself back up to starting point through a count of 10 seconds. Without resting, repeat three times. (Note: The MTP will depend on how flexible your shoulders are. Your MTP will be about an inch above your most flexible point. If this exercise is too difficult, do the Chair Dip as shown on page 69.)

ABS

EXERCISE D

Bicycle Crunch

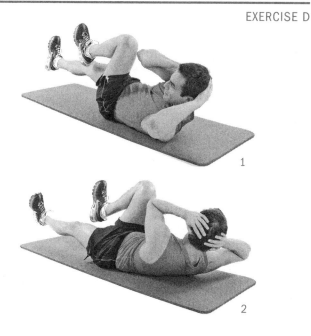

Lie flat on your back. Place your hands behind your head and raise your heels about 2 inches from the ground, keeping your chin up and abs tight throughout the exercise. Bring your right elbow to your left knee and feather your breathing as you rotate to the other side for a count of 10 seconds. Hold and squeeze for 2 seconds at the MTP (where your left elbow meets your right knee). Lower your body to starting point through a count of 10 seconds. Without resting, repeat three times.

FINISH

LEGS

Bench Squat on Cable Machine

With the pulleys on their lowest settings, stand across the bench with the bar resting across the back of your shoulders, feet slightly wider than shoulder-width apart. Keep your back straight, abs tight, and head up. Feather your breathing as you squat (as if you were about to sit at an angle on the bench) through a count of 10 seconds. Hold for 2 seconds at the MTP, about 2 inches from touching the bench. Push through your heels as you stand up and return to starting point through a count of 10 seconds. Without resting, repeat three times. **Backup move:** *Plié Squat, page 66.*

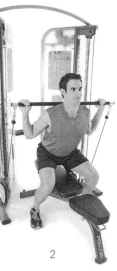

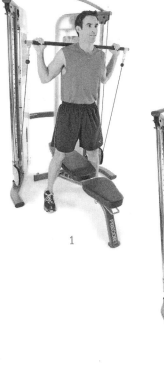

1

2

BACK

Wide-Grip Pull-down with Cable Machine

Grasp the bar attachment using a wide grip, with the pulleys on their highest settings. Sit back on your heels with your arms fully stretched. Keep your back straight, chest up, and abs tight. Feather your breathing as you pull the bar down toward the top part of your chest through a count of 10 seconds. Hold and squeeze at the MTP for 2 seconds. Resist the weight as you return it to starting point, through a count of 10 seconds. Without resting, repeat three times.

WIDE GRIP

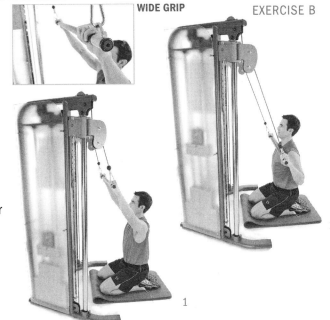

1

2

KEY: MTP: maximum tension point. **Feather your breathing:** Inhale deeply and exhale in short bursts.
Timing: Each exercise should take 90 seconds, and each circuit should take 6 minutes.

CHEST

EXERCISE C

Flat Press on Swiss Ball with Cable Machine

Lie on a Swiss ball with your head and neck supported. Grip the bar about two times wider than your shoulder width. Extend your arms and be sure to keep your back flat against the Swiss ball. Feather your breathing as you lower the bar down toward the middle of your chest through a count of 10 seconds. Hold at the MTP for 2 seconds. Press the bar up to starting point, stopping just before your elbows lock, through a count of 10 seconds. Without resting, repeat three times. **Backup move:** *Flat Press on Swiss Ball, page 79.*

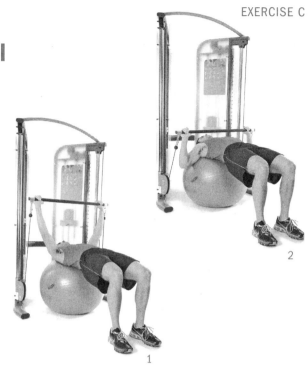

ABS

EXERCISE D

Swiss Ball Crunch with Cable Machine

With the pulley on its lowest setting, grip the rope and pull it until it is touching the back of your head. Lie on the ball and drop your hips slightly. Feather your breathing as you crunch up, pulling your elbows to your knees, through a count of 10 seconds. Hold and squeeze for 2 seconds at the MTP. Lower yourself to starting point through a count of 10 seconds. Without resting, repeat three times. **Backup move:** *Swiss Ball Crunch, page 71.*

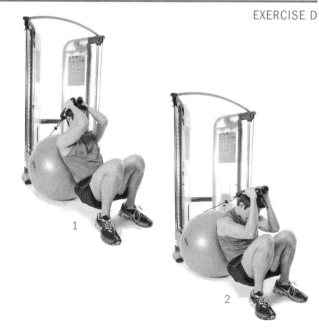

LEGS

EXERCISE A

Split Squat

Stand about 3 feet in front of a bench. Place your rear foot on the bench, with the top of your shoe lightly touching the bench. With your back straight, chest up, and abs tight, feather your breathing as you bend your front knee, lowering yourself toward the floor through a count of 10 seconds. Hold for 2 seconds at the MTP. Without resting, return to starting point through a count of 10 seconds. Repeat once more, then switch sides and perform 2 more reps, for a total of 4.

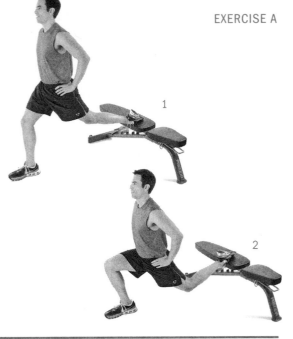

BACK

EXERCISE B

Bent-over Cable Overhand Row

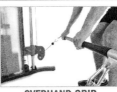

OVERHAND GRIP

Set the pulleys at their lowest setting, then grip the bar attachment using the overhand grip. Bend at the waist as if tying your shoes, and then lift only your chin and chest, creating a slight arch in your back and keeping a slight bend in your knees. Feather your breathing as you pull the bar up and back toward your hips in a rowing motion through a count of 10 seconds, keeping your elbows close to the sides of your body. Hold and squeeze your shoulder blades together at the MTP for 2 seconds. Lower the bar back to starting point through a count of 10 seconds. Without resting, repeat three times. ***Backup move:*** *Bent-over Row, page 90.*

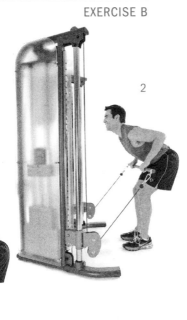

KEY: MTP: maximum tension point. **Feather your breathing:** Inhale deeply and exhale in short bursts.
Timing: Each exercise should take 90 seconds, and each circuit should take 6 minutes.

CHEST

EXERCISE C

Flat Press on Swiss Ball

Hold a pair of dumbbells and lie on the ball so that it comfortably supports your shoulder blades. Extend your arms in front of you, pressing the weights together. Feather your breathing as you lower the weights through a count of 10 seconds. Hold for 2 seconds at MTP, about 1 inch above your chest. Press the dumbbells up and together back to starting point through a count of 10 seconds. Without resting, repeat three times.

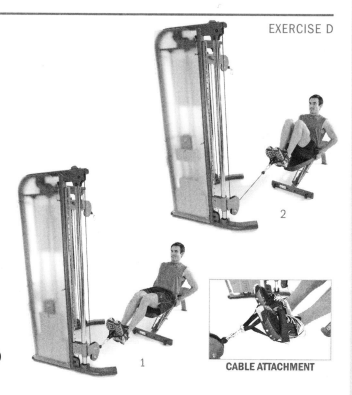

ABS

EXERCISE D

Bench Crunch (cable optional)

Sit on the edge of an exercise bench, reach your hands behind you, and grab the sides of the bench. Extend your legs forward and allow your upper body to recline back slightly. Feather your breathing as you draw your knees in and up toward your chin through a count of 10 seconds. Hold and squeeze for 2 seconds at the MTP. Return to starting point through a count of 10 seconds. Without resting, repeat three times. (For added resistance, attach your feet to the cable attachment and add a light weight.)
Backup move: *Chair Crunch, page 89.*

CABLE ATTACHMENT

LEGS

EXERCISE A

Lunge

Stand with about a 2-foot gap between your front and back leg. Keep your back straight, chest up, and abs tight. Feather your breathing as you drop your back knee toward the floor through a count of 10 seconds. Hold for 2 seconds at the MTP, about 1 inch above the ground. Return to starting position through a count of 10 seconds. Without resting, repeat one more time on this leg, then perform 2 more reps on the other side, for a total of 4 reps. (Note: To avoid injury, make sure that your front knee stays aligned with your toes and doesn't bend farther than a 90-degree angle.)

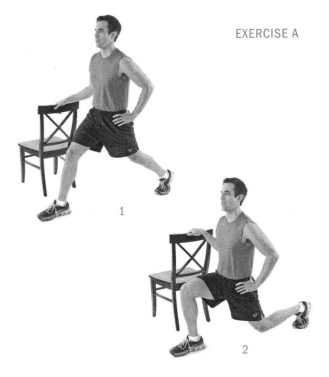

BACK

EXERCISE B

Reverse Hyperextension on Bench with Swiss Ball

With the ball on the bench, lie facedown on it. Roll yourself forward until the ball is under your hips, and your upper body is angled toward the ground. Reach forward and grip the sides of the bench for stability. With legs together, feather your breathing as you raise your heels toward the ceiling using your lower back and hamstrings. Raise through a count of 10 seconds. Hold and squeeze at the MTP for 2 seconds. With straight legs, lower through a count of 10 seconds to starting point, about 2 inches from the ground. Without resting, repeat three times. ***Backup move:*** *Reverse Hyperextension on Swiss Ball, page 104.*

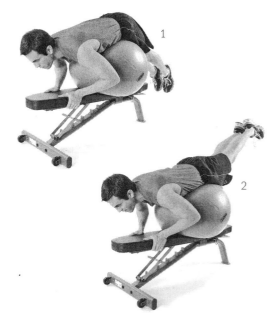

KEY: MTP: maximum tension point. **Feather your breathing:** Inhale deeply and exhale in short bursts. **Timing:** Each exercise should take 90 seconds, and each circuit should take 6 minutes.

CHEST

Downward Cable Fly

Set the pulleys on their highest settings. Grasp the handles of the pulleys after they have been set on their highest setting and take a lunge position, back straight, chest up, and abs tight. Bring your hands toward each other and press them out in front of your sternum. Feather your breathing as you slowly resist the cables out to the sides and back through a count of 10 seconds. Hold at the MTP for a count of 2 seconds. Squeeze the weight to starting point through a count of 10 seconds. Without resting, repeat three times. **Backup move:** *Flat Dumbbell Fly on Swiss Ball, page 89.*

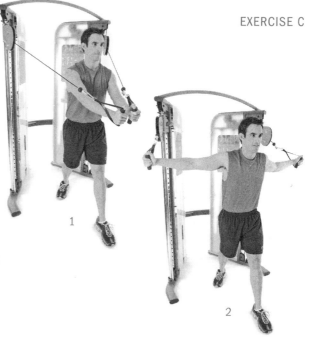

ABS

Wood Chopper on Cable Machine

With the pulley on its highest setting, grasp the handle or rope and step about 2 feet away from the machine. Place your legs about 3 feet apart; keep your chest up, back and arms straight. Feather your breathing as you pull the cable down and across your body by twisting and contracting your obliques through a count of 10 seconds. Hold and squeeze for 2 seconds at the MTP. Resist the weight to starting point, through a count of 10 seconds. Without resting, repeat once more on this side and then switch sides and complete 2 more reps. **Backup move:** *Broomstick Twist, page 67.*

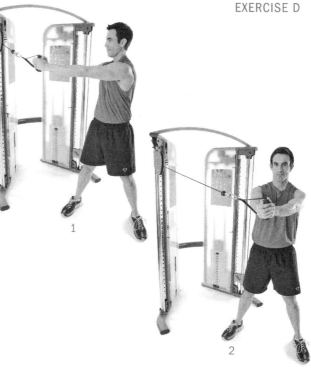

FINISH

SHOULDERS

EXERCISE A

Seated Cable Shoulder Press

Set the pulleys on their lowest setting and then grasp the bar attachment. Sit on an exercise bench or a Swiss ball. Keep your chest up, back straight, and abs tight. Pull the bar up to just under your chin. With your palms facing forward, extend the bar up over your head. Feather your breathing as you lower the bar through a count of 10 seconds. Hold the bar for 2 seconds at the MTP, just below the chin. Then press the bar to starting point through a count of 10 seconds. Without resting, repeat three times. (Note: Be sure to keep the bar in track through the movement, not too far behind or in front of you.) **Backup move:** *Shoulder Press on Swiss Ball, page 80.*

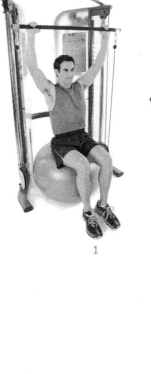

1

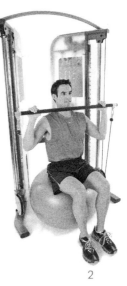

2

BICEPS

EXERCISE B

Cable Curl

Set the pulleys on their lowest settings. Hold the bar in your hands, palms facing forward and your feet shoulder-width apart, arms extended by your sides, knees slightly bent. Feather your breathing as you curl the bar up through a count of 10 seconds. Hold and squeeze for 2 seconds at the MTP. Keep your elbows tight against your body as you lower the weight through a count of 10 seconds to the starting point. Without resting, repeat three times. (Note: Be sure not to let your elbows move away from your sides throughout the entire exercise.) **Backup move:** *Standing Curl, page 68.*

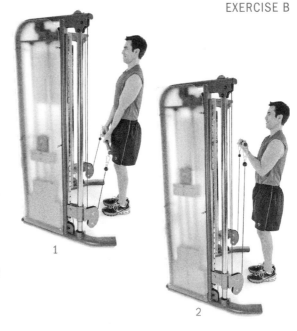

1

2

KEY: MTP: maximum tension point. **Feather your breathing:** Inhale deeply and exhale in short bursts.
Timing: Each exercise should take 90 seconds, and each circuit should take 6 minutes.

TRICEPS

Triceps Cable Press-down

Set the pulleys on their highest setting. Grasp the bar with hands about 1 foot apart. Pull your elbows against your sides and extend your arms down. Feather your breathing as you resist the bar up through a count of 10 seconds. Hold at the MTP for 2 seconds (just prior to lockout, with elbows at about a 90-degree angle). Press the weight back to starting point through a count of 10 seconds. Without resting, repeat three times. **Backup move:** *Chair Dip, page 69.*

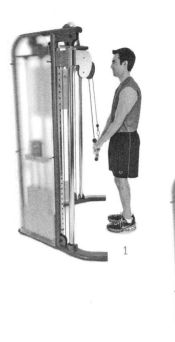

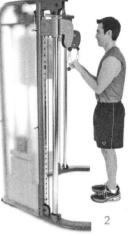

ABS

Swiss Ball Crunch with Elevated Feet

Sit on the ball about 2 feet away from a wall, arms crossed. Walk your feet out, and place them against the wall. Feather your breathing as you crunch up through a count of 10 seconds, using only your abs. Hold and squeeze for 2 seconds at the MTP. Then return to starting point through a count of 10 seconds. Without resting, repeat three times. (Note: Keep in mind that the range of motion is short on this exercise, so be sure to adjust your pace.)

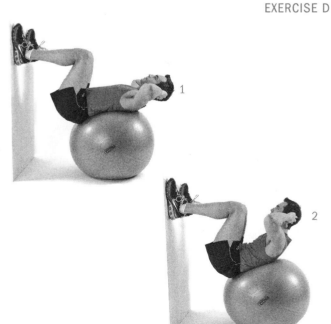

SHOULDERS

Front Delt Raise on Swiss Ball

Hold a pair of dumbbells and stand with a ball against a sturdy wall, the ball between your shoulder blades and your body slightly angled back toward the wall. Feather your breathing as you raise the dumbbells with slightly bent elbows through a count of 10 seconds. Hold for 2 seconds at the MTP (about eye level). Lower the weights back to starting point through a count of 10 seconds. Without resting, repeat three times.

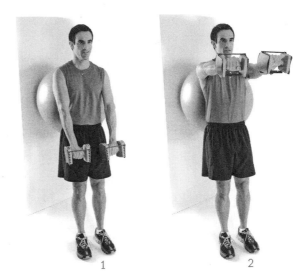

1   2

BICEPS

Incline Biceps Curl

Hold a pair of dumbbells and lie back slightly on an incline bench, allowing your arms to hang down naturally, palms facing forward. Feather your breathing as you curl the dumbbells up through a count of 10 seconds. Hold and squeeze for 2 seconds at the MTP. Lower the weights back to starting point through a count of 10 seconds, until your arm is completely straight at the bottom. Without resting, repeat three times. (Note: Be sure not to let the elbows move away from your body.)

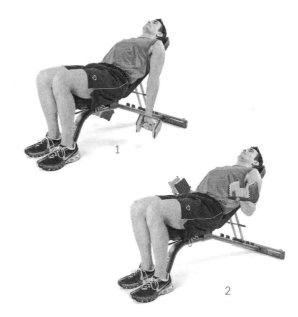

1

2

KEY: MTP: maximum tension point. **Feather your breathing:** Inhale deeply and exhale in short bursts.
Timing: Each exercise should take 90 seconds, and each circuit should take 6 minutes.

TRICEPS

EXERCISE C

Bench Dip on Swiss Ball

Sit on the front edge of a sturdy chair or exercise bench, hands close by your sides, fingers forward, and legs extended on a Swiss ball. Feather your breathing as you lower yourself through a count of 10 seconds. Hold at the MTP for 2 seconds. Push yourself back up to starting point through a count of 10 seconds. Without resting, repeat three times. (Note: The MTP will depend on how flexible your shoulders are. Your MTP will be about an inch above your most flexible point. If this exercise is too difficult, do the Chair Dip as shown on page 69.

ABS

EXERCISE D

Knees to Elbows on Bench

Lie close to the upper end of the bench. Reach behind you and grab the bench next to your ears. Squeeze your elbows together and keep your chin up and abs tight. Feather your breathing as you pull your knees up slowly to your elbows through a count of 10 seconds. Hold and squeeze for 2 seconds at the MTP (where the elbows touch the knees). Return to starting point through a count of 10 seconds, never letting your feet touch the ground. Without resting, repeat three times.

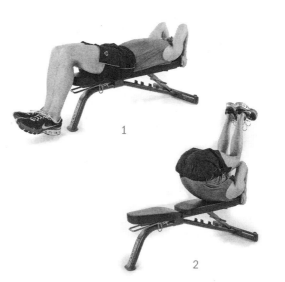

SHOULDERS

Rear Delt Cable Extension

EXERCISE A

Adjust the pulleys so that they are at shoulder level. Using the handles, cross your arms and grasp the cables, then step back until your hands are on top of one another. Feather your breathing as you extend your arms back to a "T" position through a count of 10 seconds. Hold and squeeze at the MTP for a count of 2 seconds. Resist the cables back to starting point through a count of 10 seconds. Without resting, repeat three times. **Backup move:** *Seated Rear Delt Raise, page 72.*

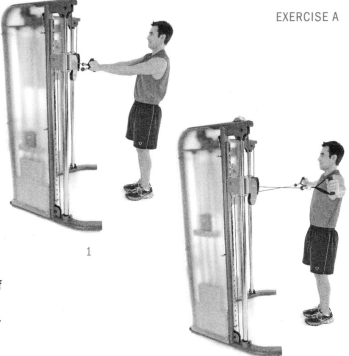

1

2

BICEPS

EXERCISE B

Reclined Cable Bar Curl

Set the pulleys to their lowest settings. Grip the bar attachment and sit back on an incline bench, palms facing upward, keeping your elbows by your sides, arms fully extended. Feather your breathing as you curl the bar up toward your deltoids through a count of 10 seconds. Hold and squeeze at the MTP (where the biceps are at full contraction) for 2 seconds. Lower the bar down to starting point through a count of 10 seconds. Without resting, repeat three times. (Note: Be sure not to let your elbows drift away from your sides at any point throughout the exercise.) **Backup move:** *Standing Curl, page 68.*

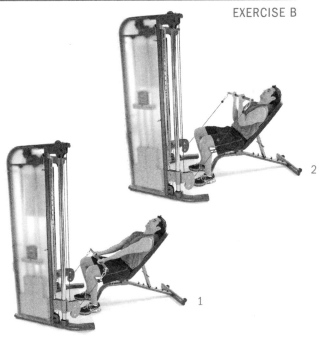

2

1

KEY: MTP: maximum tension point. **Feather your breathing:** Inhale deeply and exhale in short bursts.
Timing: Each exercise should take 90 seconds, and each circuit should take 6 minutes.

TRICEPS

Overhead Triceps Cable Extension

Set the pulleys on their lowest settings. Grip the bar attachment with your palms facing upward, and sit against the ball with your chest up and abs tight. Extend your arms, keeping your biceps tight against your head. Feather your breathing as you lower the bar down behind your head through a count of 10 seconds. Hold for 2 seconds at the MTP (when the elbow is at a 90-degree angle). Extend the bar to starting point through a count of 10 seconds. Without resting, repeat three times. (Note: Avoid letting your elbows drift outward or arching your back throughout this exercise.) ***Backup move:*** *Overhead Triceps Extension on Swiss Ball, page 81.*

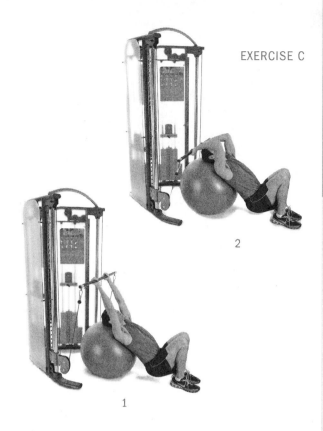

ABS

Oblique Side Bends on Roman Chair

Cross your arms and lie on your side in the Roman chair. Lean down to begin the exercise. Keeping your back straight and abs tight, crunch up through a count of 10 seconds. Hold and squeeze at the MTP for 2 seconds. Lower yourself down through a count of 10 seconds. Without resting, repeat once more on this side and then switch sides and complete 2 more reps.

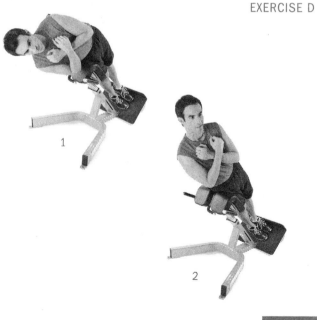

FINISH

LEGS

EXERCISE A

Split Squat

Stand about 3 feet in front of a bench. Place your rear foot on the bench, with the top of your shoe lightly touching the bench. With your back straight, chest up, and abs tight, feather your breathing as you bend your front knee, lowering yourself toward the ground through a count of 10 seconds. Hold for 2 seconds at the MTP. Without resting, return back to starting point through a count of 10 seconds. Repeat once more, then switch sides and perform 2 more reps, for a total of 4.

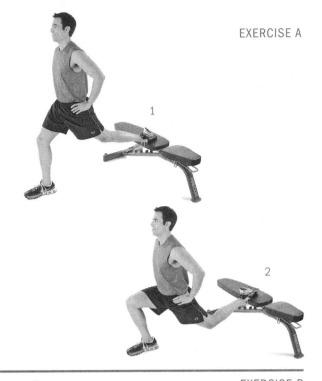

BACK

EXERCISE B

Close-Grip Pull-down on Cable Machine

Grasp a close-grip handle with the pulley on its highest setting. Sit back onto your heels with your arms fully stretched; keep your back straight, chest up, and abs tight. Feather your breathing as you pull the handle down toward the top part of your chest through a count of 10 seconds. Hold and squeeze at the MTP for 2 seconds. Lower the weight to starting point through a count of 10 seconds. Without resting, repeat three times.

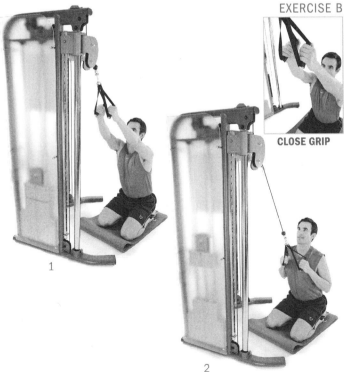

CLOSE GRIP

KEY: MTP: maximum tension point. **Feather your breathing:** Inhale deeply and exhale in short bursts.
Timing: Each exercise should take 90 seconds, and each circuit should take 6 minutes.

CHEST

Incline Cable Barbell Press on Swiss Ball

Set the pulleys to their lowest setting. Grip the bar about two times wider than your shoulder width, and lie on the ball so that your head and neck are supported. Allow your hips to drop almost to the ground. Extend your arms and be sure to keep your back pressed against the ball. Feather your breathing as you lower the bar down toward the top of your sternum through a count of 10 seconds. Hold for 2 seconds at the MTP. Press the bar up to starting point (just prior to lockout) through a count of 10 seconds. Without resting, repeat three times.
Backup move: *Incline Press on Swiss Ball, page 63.*

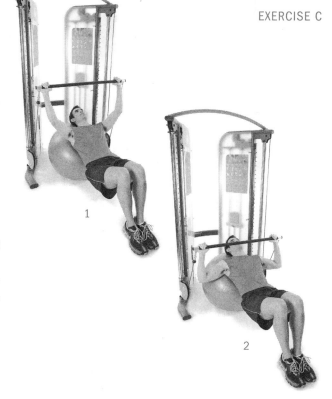

ABS

Swiss Ball Crunch with Cable Machine

With the pulley on its lowest setting, grip the rope and pull it until it is touching the back of your head. Lie on the ball and drop your hips down slightly. Feather your breathing as you crunch up, pulling your elbows to your knees, through a count of 10 seconds. Hold and squeeze for 2 seconds at the MTP. Lower yourself to starting point through a count of 10 seconds. Without resting, repeat three times. **Backup move:** *Swiss Ball Crunch, page 71.*

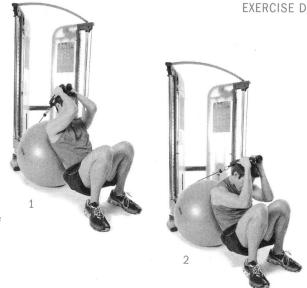

LEGS

Bench Squat on Cable Machine

With the pulleys on their lowest settings, straddle the bench with the bar resting across the back of your shoulders, feet slightly wider than shoulder-width apart. Keep your back straight, abs tight, and head up. Feather your breathing as you squat down (as if you were about to sit at an angle on the bench) through a count of 10 seconds. Hold for 2 seconds at the MTP, about 2 inches from touching the bench. Push through your heels as you stand up and return to starting point through a count of 10 seconds. Without resting, repeat three times. **Backup move:** *Plié Squat, page 66.*

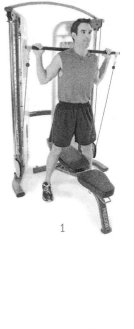

1

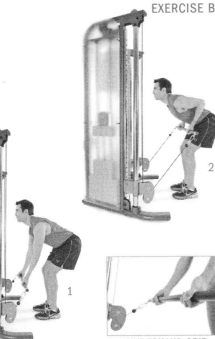

2

BACK

Bent-over Row on Cable Machine (underhand grip)

With the pulleys on their lowest settings, hold the bar using the underhand grip. Bend at the waist as if tying your shoes, and then lift only your chin and chest, creating a slight arch in the back while keeping a slight bend in your knees. Feather your breathing as you pull the bar up and back toward your hips through a count of 10 seconds, keeping your elbows close to the sides of your body. Hold and squeeze your shoulder blades together at the MTP for 2 seconds. Lower the bar back to starting position through a count of 10 seconds. Without resting, repeat three times. **Backup move:** *Bent-over Row (underhand grip), page 76.*

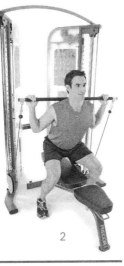

2

1

UNDERHAND GRIP

KEY: MTP: maximum tension point. **Feather your breathing:** Inhale deeply and exhale in short bursts.
Timing: Each exercise should take 90 seconds, and each circuit should take 6 minutes.

CHEST

Incline Dumbbell Press

Hold a pair of dumbbells and lie back on the bench. Press the weights up and together, with a slight bend in the elbows, keeping your back straight and abs tight. Feather your breathing as you lower the weights through a count of 10 seconds. Hold for 2 seconds at the MTP. Press the dumbbells up to starting point through a count of 10 seconds. Without resting, repeat three times.

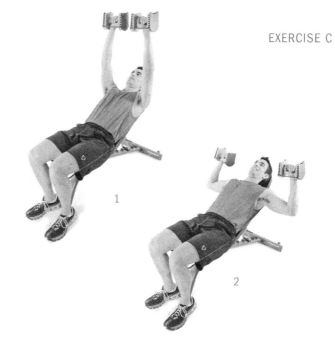

ABS

Double Crunch on Bench

Lie on a flat bench with a dumbbell under your chin for added resistance. Raise your feet off the ground about 2 inches. Feather your breathing as you simultaneously crunch and raise your knees through a count of 10 seconds. Hold and squeeze for 2 seconds at the MTP. Return to starting point through a count of 10 seconds. Be sure to keep your feet 2 inches from the ground at the bottom of the motion. Without resting, repeat three times.

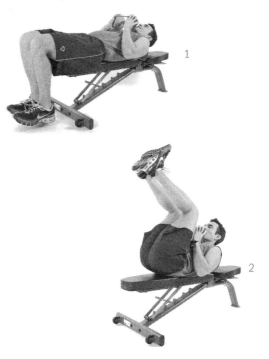

LEGS

Hamstring Kickback on Bench (cable optional)

Attach the cable to the ankle attachment. Place one knee on the bench while using both hands to support your weight. Keep your head up and back straight throughout the exercise, and your foot flexed. Feather your breathing as you lift one leg up and back through a count of 10 seconds, keeping your leg locked. Hold and squeeze for 2 seconds at the MTP. Return to starting point through a count of 10 seconds. Without resting, repeat once more, then switch sides and complete 2 more, for a total of 4 reps. **Backup move:** *Glute Kickback on Swiss Ball, page 78.*

EXERCISE A

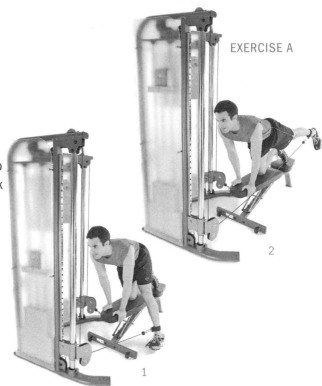

BACK

EXERCISE B

Hyperextension on Roman Chair

Position yourself on a Roman chair with your arms crossed in front of you. Bend at the waist. Feather your breathing as you raise your upper body through a count of 10 seconds. Hold and squeeze for 2 seconds at the MTP. Lower to starting position through a count of 10. Without resting, repeat three times. (Note: The MTP will vary depending on your level of flexibility.)

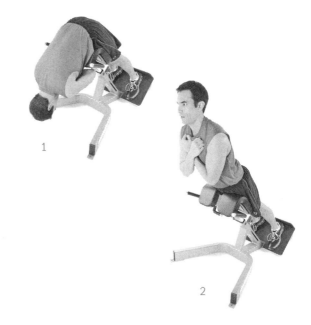

KEY: MTP: maximum tension point. **Feather your breathing:** Inhale deeply and exhale in short bursts.
Timing: Each exercise should take 90 seconds, and each circuit should take 6 minutes.

CHEST

Upward Cable Fly

Set the pulleys on their lowest settings. Grasp the handles with palms facing outward and take a lunge position. Feather your breathing as you raise the cables, squeezing them together throughout the movement. Hold and squeeze at the MTP for a count of 2 seconds. Resist the weight back to its starting position through a count of 10 seconds. Without resting, repeat three times. ***Backup move:*** *Incline Dumbbell Fly on Swiss Ball, page 77.*

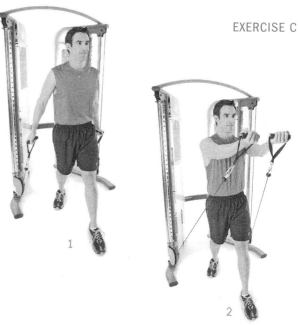

ABS

Cable Russian Twist on Ball

Set the pulley about waist level. Grasp the handle attachment and lie on the ball with your head and neck supported keeping your hips up, arms straight, and abs tight. Feather your breathing as you rotate your torso through a count of 10 seconds. Hold and squeeze for 2 seconds at the MTP (when your arms are about parallel to the floor). Rotate back to starting point through a count of 10 seconds. Without resting, alternate sides and complete 2 reps on each side for a total of 4. ***Backup move:*** *Russian Twist, page 85.*

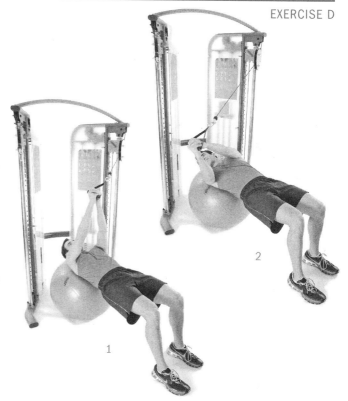

FINISH

SHOULDERS

Seated Cable Shoulder Press

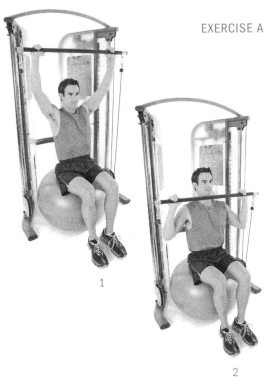

EXERCISE A

Grasp the bar attachment with the pulleys on their lowest settings, palms facing forward. Sit back into the upright bench or on the ball. Keep your chest up, back straight, and abs tight. Pull the bar up to just under your chin. Extend the bar up over your head and feather your breathing as you lower the bar through a count of 10 seconds. Hold the bar for 2 seconds at the MTP, just below the chin. Press the bar to starting point through a count of 10 seconds. Without resting, repeat three times. (Note: Be sure to keep the bar in track through the movement, not too far behind or in front of you.) **Backup move:** *Shoulder Press on Swiss Ball, page 80.*

BICEPS

EXERCISE B

Standing Biceps Cable Curl

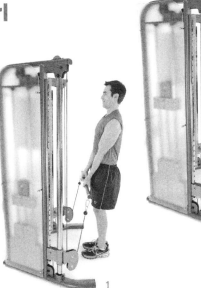

Begin by grasping the bar attachment with the pulleys on their lowest settings. Stand with your feet about shoulder-width apart with a 10- to 12-inch space between your hands. With your arms extended and elbows tight by your sides, feather your breathing as you curl the bar up through a count of 10 seconds. Hold and squeeze at the MTP for 2 seconds (where the biceps are fully contracted). Lower the bar down to starting point through a count of 10 seconds. Without resting, repeat three times. (Note: Be sure not to let your elbows drift away from your sides at any point throughout the exercise.) **Backup move:** *Standing Curl, page 106.*

KEY: MTP: maximum tension point. **Feather your breathing:** Inhale deeply and exhale in short bursts.
Timing: Each exercise should take 90 seconds, and each circuit should take 6 minutes.

TRICEPS

EXERCISE C

Cable "Skull Crusher" on Swiss Ball with Rope

With the pulley on its lowest setting, grasp the rope and lie on the ball so that your head and neck are supported. Keep your hips up and abs tight throughout the exercise. Extend the rope with a slight bend in your elbows, palms facing each other. Drop your arms back slightly, about 2 inches, and feather your breathing as you bend your elbows and lower the weight down through a count of 10 seconds. Hold at the MTP for 2 seconds, about an inch above your forehead. Raise the weight back to starting point through a count of 10 seconds. Without resting, repeat three times. **Backup move:** *Dumbbell "Skull Crusher" on Swiss Ball, page 71.*

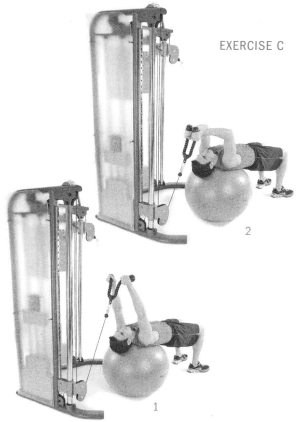

ABS

EXERCISE D

Knees to Elbows on Bench

Lie close to the end of the bench. Reach behind you and grab the bench next to your ears. Squeeze your elbows together and keep your chin up and abs tight. Feather your breathing as you pull your knees up slowly to your elbows through a count of 10 seconds. Hold and squeeze for 2 seconds at the MTP (where the elbows touch the knees). Return to starting point through a count of 10 seconds, never letting your feet touch the ground. Without resting, repeat three times.

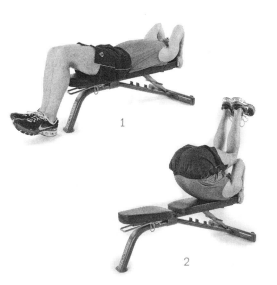

SHOULDERS

Standing Cable Lateral Raise

With the pulleys set at about shoulder level, grasp the handles using the cross grip. Stand upright, keeping your abs tight and back straight. Feather your breathing as you raise the handles up through a count of 10 seconds. Hold and squeeze for 2 seconds at the MTP. Then lower the weight to starting point, through a count of 10 seconds. Without resting, repeat three times. **Backup move:** *Standing Lateral Raise, page 70.*

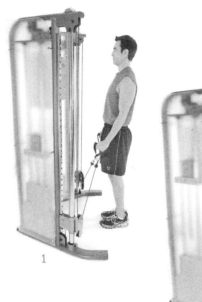

BICEPS

Standing Side Curl

Hold a pair of dumbbells with your palms turned out, elbows to your sides. Keep your chest up, feet hip-width apart, knees slightly bent, and abs tight throughout the exercise. Feather your breathing as you curl the weights up through a count of 10 seconds. Hold and squeeze at the MTP for a count of 2 seconds, then lower the weights to starting point through a count of 10 seconds until your arms are nearly straight (do not lock your elbows). Without resting, repeat three times. (Note: As you perform the exercise, be sure to keep your elbows tight against your body.)

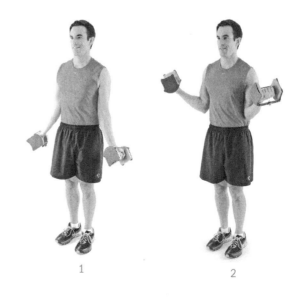

KEY: MTP: maximum tension point. **Feather your breathing:** Inhale deeply and exhale in short bursts. **Timing:** Each exercise should take 90 seconds, and each circuit should take 6 minutes.

TRICEPS

Triceps Cable Press-down

Set the pulleys on their highest setting. Grasp the bar with hands about 1 foot apart. Pull your elbows against your sides and extend your arms downward. Feather your breathing as you resist the bar up through a count of 10 seconds. Hold at the MTP for 2 seconds (just prior to lockout, with elbows at about a 90-degree angle). Press the weight back to starting point through a count of 10 seconds. Without resting, repeat three times. **Backup move:** *Chair Dip, page 69.*

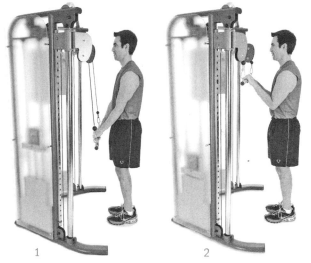

1   2

ABS

Swiss Ball Crunch with Cable Machine

With the pulley on its lowest setting, grip the rope and pull it until it is touching the back of your head. Lie on the ball and drop your hips down slightly. Feather your breathing as you crunch up, pulling your elbows to your knees, through a count of 10 seconds. Hold and squeeze for 2 seconds at the MTP. Lower yourself to starting point through a count of 10 seconds. Without resting, repeat three times. **Backup move:** *Swiss Ball Crunch, page 71.*

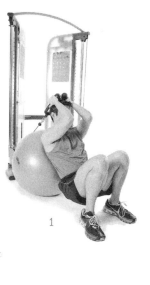

1

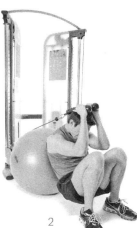

2

SHOULDERS

Reclined Rear Delt Cable Extension

With the pulleys on their highest settings, grasp the handles using a cross grip and lie back on the inclined bench. Extend your arms and slightly bend your elbows. Feather your breathing as you pull your arms back in an "arch" motion through a count of 10 seconds. Hold and squeeze for 2 seconds at the MTP. Return to starting point through a count of 10 seconds. Without resting, repeat three times. ***Backup move:*** *Seated Rear Delt Raise, page 72.*

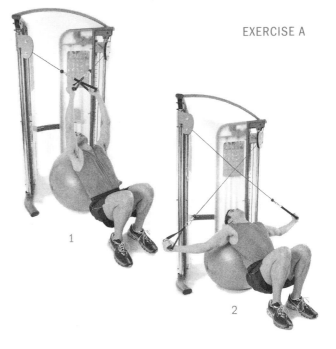

BICEPS

Cable Preacher Curl on Swiss Ball

Begin by setting the bar attachment with the pulleys on their lowest settings. Lean over the ball with your knees on the floor and grab the bar, hands about 1 foot apart, palms facing up. Feather your breathing as you curl the weight up through a count of 10 seconds. Hold and squeeze at the MTP for a count of 2 seconds. Lower the weight to starting point through a count of 10 seconds. Without resting, repeat three times. (Note: The preacher curl is the only curl in which you shouldn't allow your arms to extend fully. Keep them slightly bent at the bottom of the motion.) ***Backup move:*** *Preacher Curl on Swiss Ball, page 72.*

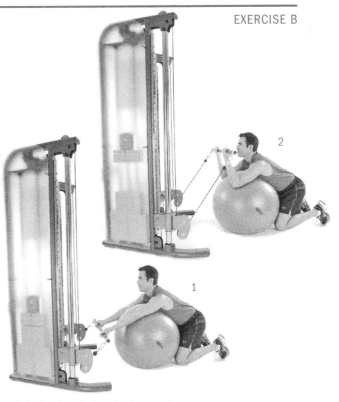

KEY: MTP: maximum tension point. **Feather your breathing:** Inhale deeply and exhale in short bursts.
Timing: Each exercise should take 90 seconds, and each circuit should take 6 minutes.

TRICEPS

Overhead Triceps Cable Extension

Set the pulleys on their lowest settings. Grip the bar attachment with your palms facing the ceiling, and sit on the incline bench with your chest up and abs tight. Extend your arms, keeping your biceps tight against your head. Feather your breathing as you lower the bar behind your head through a count of 10 seconds. Hold for 2 seconds at the MTP (when the elbow is at a 90-degree angle). Extend the bar to starting point through a count of 10 seconds. Without resting, repeat three times. (Note: Avoid letting your elbows drift outward or arching your back throughout this exercise.) ***Backup move:*** *Overhead Triceps Extension on Swiss Ball, page 81.*

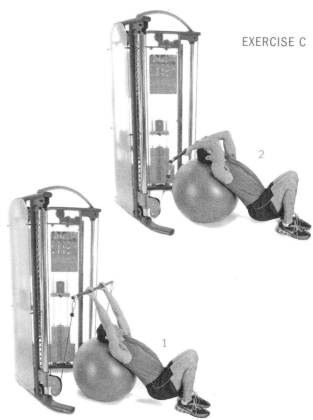

ABS

Jackknife

Begin standing about 3 feet in front of the ball, and place your palms on the ground, hands shoulder-width apart. From here put one foot on the ball about mid-shin level. Once level, place the other foot on the ball, keeping your head forward, spine straight, and abs tight. Slowly pull your knees up to your chin through a count of 10 seconds, as you concentrate on keeping stability by squeezing your abs tight. Hold and squeeze for 2 seconds at the MTP. Return to starting point through a count of 10 seconds. Without resting, repeat three times.

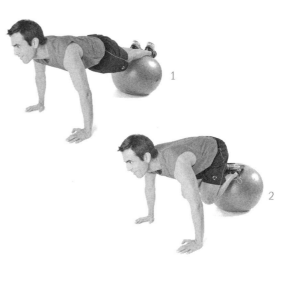

LEGS

Bench Squat on Cable Machine

With the pulleys on their lowest settings, straddle the bench with the bar resting across the back of your shoulders, feet slightly wider than shoulder-width apart. Keep your back straight, abs tight, and head up. Feather your breathing as you squat (as if you were about to sit at an angle on the bench) through a count of 10 seconds. Hold for 2 seconds at the MTP, about 2 inches from touching the bench. Push through your heels as you stand up and return to starting point through a count of 10 seconds. Without resting, repeat three times. **Backup move:** *Plié Squat, page 66.*

EXERCISE A

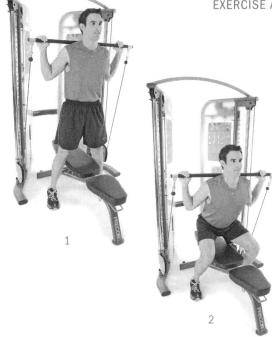

BACK

EXERCISE B

Pull-down on Cable Machine (underhand grip)

With the pulleys on their highest settings, grasp the bar attachment using the underhand grip. Sit back onto your heels with your arms fully stretched; keep your back straight, chest up, and abs tight. Feather your breathing as you pull the bar down toward the top part of your chest through a count of 10 seconds. Hold and squeeze at the MTP for 2 seconds. Then lower the weight to starting point through a count of 10 seconds. Without resting, repeat three times.

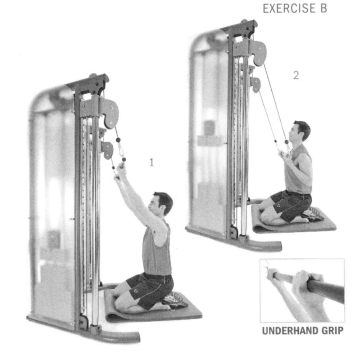

UNDERHAND GRIP

KEY: MTP: maximum tension point. **Feather your breathing:** Inhale deeply and exhale in short bursts.
Timing: Each exercise should take 90 seconds, and each circuit should take 6 minutes.

CHEST

Cable Flat Barbell Press on Swiss Ball

With the pulleys on their lowest settings, grip the bar attachment and lie on the ball with your hips elevated. Press the bar up over your chest with your elbows slightly bent. Feather your breathing as you lower the bar to your chest through a count of 10 seconds. Hold for 2 seconds at the MTP. Press the bar, returning to starting point through a count of 10 seconds. Without resting, repeat three times. **Backup move:** *Flat Press on Swiss Ball, page 79.*

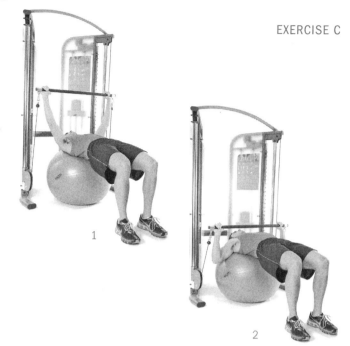

ABS

Jackknife

Begin standing about 3 feet in front of the ball, and place your palms on the ground, hands shoulder-width apart. From here put one foot on the ball about mid-shin level. Once level, place the other foot on the ball, keeping your head forward, spine straight, and abs tight. Slowly pull your knees up to your chin through a count of 10 seconds, as you concentrate on maintaining stability by squeezing your abs tight. Hold and squeeze 2 seconds at the MTP. Return to starting point through a count of 10 seconds. Without resting, repeat three times.

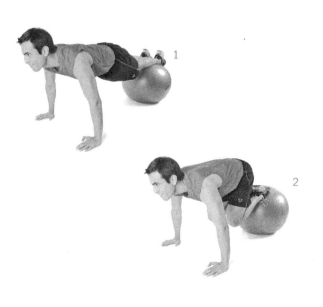

LEGS

Split Squat

Stand about 3 feet in front of a bench. Place your rear foot on the bench, with the top of your shoe lightly touching the bench. With your back straight, chest up, and abs tight, feather your breathing as you bend your front knee, lowering yourself toward the floor through a count of 10 seconds. Hold for 2 seconds at the MTP. Without resting, return to starting point through a count of 10 seconds. Repeat once more, then switch sides and perform 2 more reps, for a total of 4.

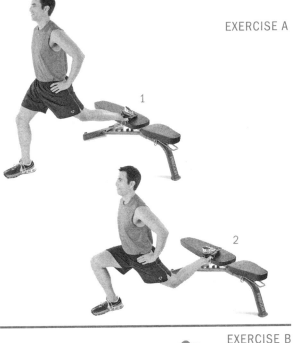

EXERCISE A

BACK

Bent-over Cable Row (close grip)

With the pulley at is lowest setting, grasp the close-grip handle. Bend at the waist as if tying your shoes, and lift only your chin and chest, creating a slight arch in your back. Keep a slight bend in your knees and feather your breathing as you pull the handle up and back to your hips through a count of 10 seconds. Hold and squeeze your shoulder blades together for 2 seconds at the MTP. Lower the dumbbells back to starting position through a count of 10 seconds. Without resting, repeat three times. (Note: Keep your elbows close to the sides of your body.) ***Backup move:*** *Bent-over Row (standard grip), page 90.*

EXERCISE B

CLOSE GRIP

KEY: MTP: maximum tension point. **Feather your breathing:** Inhale deeply and exhale in short bursts.
Timing: Each exercise should take 90 seconds, and each circuit should take 6 minutes.

CHEST

EXERCISE C

Flat Press on Swiss Ball

Hold a pair of dumbbells and lie on the ball so that it comfortably supports your shoulder blades. Extend your arms in front of you, pressing the weights together. Feather your breathing as you lower the weights through a count of 10 seconds. Hold for 2 seconds at the MTP, about 1 inch above your chest. Press the dumbbells up and together back to starting point through a count of 10 seconds. Without resting, repeat three times.

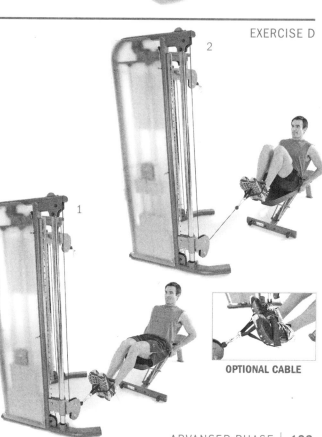

ABS

EXERCISE D

Bench Crunch (cable optional)

Sitting on the edge of an exercise bench, reach your hands behind you and grab the sides of the bench. Extend your legs forward and allow your upper body to recline back slightly. Feather your breathing as you draw your knees in and up toward your chin through a count of 10 seconds. Hold and squeeze for 2 seconds at the MTP. Return to starting point through a count of 10 seconds. Without resting, repeat three times. (For added resistance, attach your feet to the cable attachment and add a light weight.)

OPTIONAL CABLE

LEGS

Lateral Squat

Take a stance about a foot wider than shoulder-width on each side. Feather your breathing as you squat toward one leg while keeping the opposite leg straight, through a count of 10 seconds. Hold for 2 seconds at the MTP. Return to starting point through a count of 10 seconds. Without resting, alternate sides and complete 2 reps on each side for a total of 4.

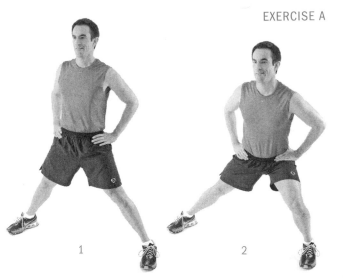

BACK

Dumbbell Dead Lift

Stand holding a dumbbell in each hand, with your feet about 6 to 8 inches apart. Bend forward from the hips as if you were about to tie your shoes. Lift your chin and chest, creating a slight arch in your back. Feather your breathing as you lift your upper body through a count of 10, driving through your heels and using your lower back and hamstrings. Hold for 2 seconds at the MTP (at the top of the movement). Return to starting position through a count of 10 seconds. Without resting, repeat three times.

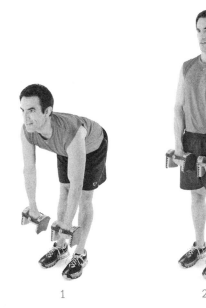

KEY: MTP: maximum tension point. **Feather your breathing:** Inhale deeply and exhale in short bursts.
Timing: Each exercise should take 90 seconds, and each circuit should take 6 minutes.

CHEST

EXERCISE C

Downward Cable Fly

Set the pulleys on their highest settings. Grasp the handles of the pulleys and take a lunge position, back straight, chest up, and abs tight. Bring your hands toward each other and press them out in front of your sternum. Feather your breathing as you slowly resist the cables out to the sides and back through a count of 10 seconds. Hold at the MTP for a count of 2 seconds. Squeeze the weight back to starting point through a count of 10 seconds. Without resting, repeat three times. **Backup move:** *Flat Dumbbell Fly on Swiss Ball, page 67.*

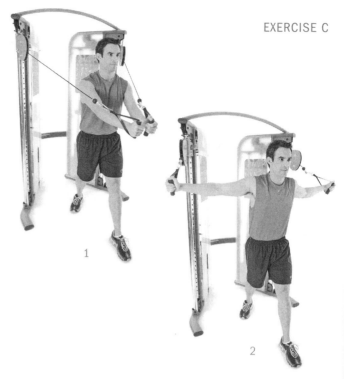

ABS

EXERCISE D

Bicycle Crunch

Lie flat on your back. Place your hands behind your head and raise your heels about 2 inches from the ground, keeping your chin up and abs tight throughout the exercise. Bring your right elbow toward your left knee and feather your breathing as you rotate to the other side for a count of 10 seconds. Hold and squeeze for 2 seconds at the MTP (where the elbow meets the knee). Lower to starting position through a count of 10 seconds. Without resting, repeat three times.

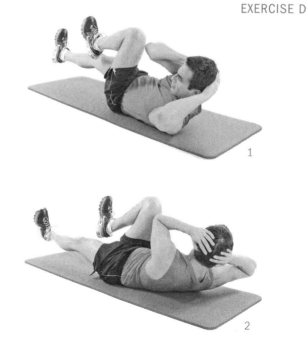

FINISH

SHOULDERS

EXERCISE A

Seated Shoulder Press on Bench

Hold a pair of dumbbells and sit on an upright bench. With your palms facing forward, extend the weights up over your head. Feather your breathing as you lower the weights through a count of 10 seconds. Hold and squeeze for 2 seconds at the MTP (chin level). Press the weight up to starting point through a count of 10 seconds. Without resting, repeat three times.

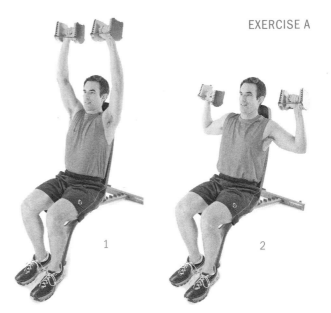

1

2

BICEPS

EXERCISE B

Standing Curl

Hold a pair of dumbbells and stand with your feet shoulder-width apart and your arms extended by your sides, with your palms facing forward and your knees slightly bent. Feather your breathing as you curl the dumbbells up through a count of 10 seconds to just past a 90-degree angle. Hold and squeeze for 2 seconds at the MTP, then lower the weights to starting point through a count of 10 seconds. Without resting, repeat three times. (Note: Keep the elbows tight against your sides throughout the entire exercise.)

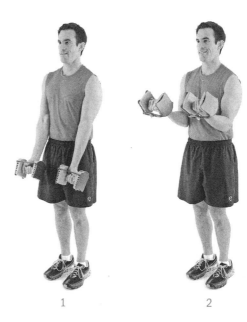

1

2

KEY: MTP: maximum tension point. **Feather your breathing:** Inhale deeply and exhale in short bursts.
Timing: Each exercise should take 90 seconds, and each circuit should take 6 minutes.

TRICEPS

Triceps Cable Pressdown with Rope

Grasp the rope with the pulley on its highest setting, palms facing each other. Hold your elbows against your sides and lower the rope to a position about even with your chest. Feather your breathing as you pull the rope down through a count of 10 seconds, rotating your hands out at the end of the motion. Hold and squeeze at the MTP (just prior to lockout) for 2 seconds. Resist the weight back to starting point through a count of 10 seconds. Without resting, repeat three times. **Backup move:** *Chair Dip, page 69.*

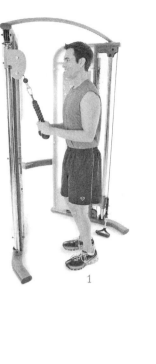

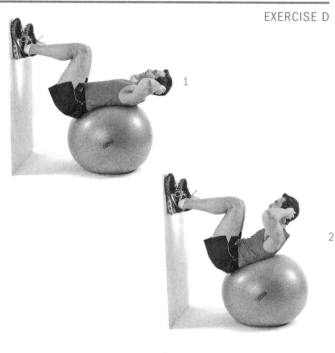

ABS

Swiss Ball Crunch with Elevated Feet

Sit on the ball about 2 feet away from a wall, hands behind your head. Walk your feet out and place them against the wall. Feather your breathing as you crunch up through a count of 10 seconds, using only your abs. Hold and squeeze for 2 seconds at the MTP. Return to starting point through a count of 10 seconds. Without resting, repeat three times. (Note: The range of motion is short on this exercise, so be sure to adjust your pace.)

SHOULDER

Upright Cable Row

With the pulleys on their lowest settings, grasp the bar attachment with an 8-inch gap between your hands, palms facing your body. Stand upright with your back straight and abs tight. Feather your breathing as you raise the bar to your chin through a count of 10 seconds. Hold and squeeze for 2 seconds at the MTP. Lower the weight back to starting point through a count of 10 seconds. Without resting, repeat three times.
Backup move: *Upright Row, page 108.*

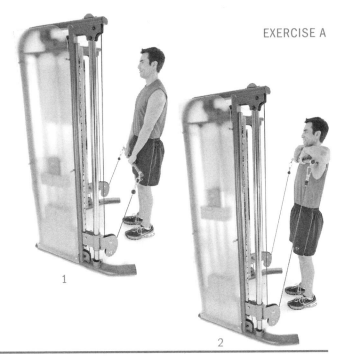

BICEPS

Incline Biceps Curl

Hold a pair of dumbbells and sit back into an incline bench, allowing your arms to hang down naturally, palms facing forward. Feather your breathing as you curl the dumbbells up through a count of 10 seconds. Hold and squeeze for 2 seconds at the MTP. Lower the weights back to starting point through a count of 10 seconds, until your arms are completely straight at the bottom (do not lock your elbows). Without resting, repeat three times. (Note: Keep your elbows tight against your body throughout the exercise.)

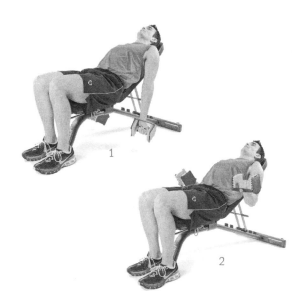

KEY: MTP: maximum tension point. **Feather your breathing:** Inhale deeply and exhale in short bursts.
Timing: Each exercise should take 90 seconds, and each circuit should take 6 minutes.

TRICEPS

EXERCISE C

Bench Dip with Swiss Ball

Sit on the front edge of a bench, hands close by your sides, fingers forward, legs extended on the ball. Feather your breathing as you lower yourself through a count of 10 seconds. Hold at the MTP for 2 seconds. Push yourself back up to starting point through a count of 10 seconds. Without resting, repeat three times. (Note: The MTP will depend on how flexible your shoulders are. Your MTP will be about an inch above your most flexible point. If this exercise is too difficult, do the Chair Dip as shown on page 69.)

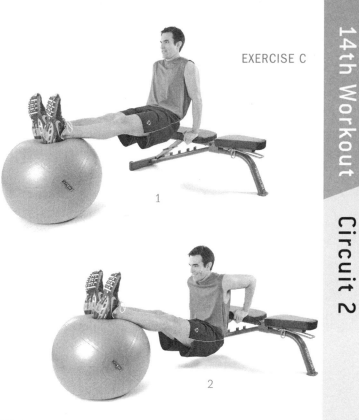

ABS

EXERCISE D

Double Crunch on Bench

Lie on a flat bench with a dumbbell under your chin for added resistance. Raise your feet off the ground about 2 inches. Feather your breathing as you simultaneously crunch and raise your knees up through a count of 10 seconds. Hold and squeeze for 2 seconds at the MTP. Return to starting position through a count of 10 seconds. Be sure to keep your feet 2 inches from the ground at the bottom of the motion. Without resting, repeat three times.

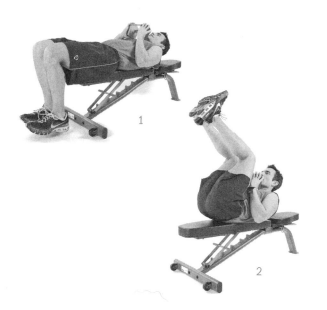

SHOULDERS

Rear Delt Cable Extension

Adjust the pulleys so that they are at shoulder level. Using the handles, cross your arms and grasp the cables, then step back until your hands are on top of one another. Feather your breathing as you extend your arms back to a "T" position through a count of 10 seconds. Hold and squeeze at the MTP for a count of 2 seconds. Resist the cables back to starting point through a count of 10 seconds. Without resting, repeat three times. **Backup move:** *Seated Rear Delt Raise, page 72.*

EXERCISE A

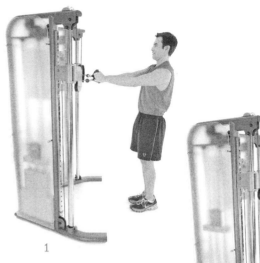

BICEPS

Reclined Cable Bar Curl

Grip the bar attachment with the pulleys on their lowest settings. Sit back into the incline bench, keeping your elbows by your sides, arms fully extended. Feather your breathing as you curl the bar up through a count of 10 seconds. Hold and squeeze at the MTP (where the biceps are at full contraction) for 2 seconds. Lower the bar down to starting point through a count of 10 seconds. Without resting, repeat three times. (Note: Keep your elbows tight against your body throughout the exercise.) **Backup move:** *Standing Curl, page 68.*

EXERCISE B

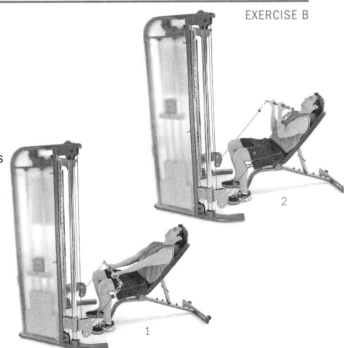

KEY: MTP: maximum tension point. **Feather your breathing:** Inhale deeply and exhale in short bursts.
Timing: Each exercise should take 90 seconds, and each circuit should take 6 minutes.

TRICEPS

Cable "Skull Crusher" on Swiss Ball with Rope

With the pulley on its lowest setting, grasp the rope and lie on the ball so that your head and neck are supported. Keep your hips up and abs tight throughout the exercise. Extend the rope with a slight bend in your elbows, palms facing each other. Drop your arms back slightly, about 2 inches, and feather your breathing as you bend your elbows and lower the weight through a count of 10. Hold at the MTP for 2 seconds, about an inch above your forehead. Raise the weight back to starting point through a count of 10. Without resting, repeat three times. ***Backup move:*** *Dumbbell "Skull Crusher" on Swiss Ball, page 71.*

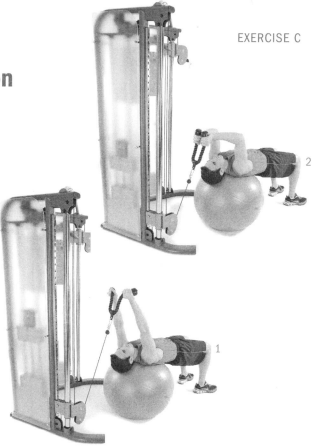

ABS

Oblique Side Bends on Roman Chair

Cross your arms and lie on your side on the Roman chair. Lean down to begin the exercise. Keep your back straight and abs tight. Crunch up through a count of 10 seconds. Hold and squeeze at the MTP for 2 seconds. Lower yourself through a count of 10 seconds. Without resting, repeat once more on this side, then switch sides and complete 2 more reps, for a total of 4 reps.

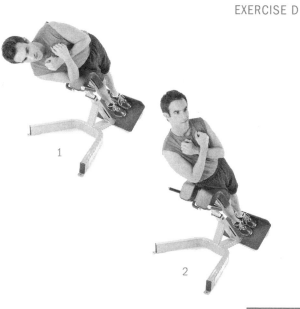

FINISH

LEGS

EXERCISE A

Plié Squat

Hold one dumbbell with both hands and stand with your feet about twice shoulder-width apart, toes turned out to the sides aligning with knees. Feather your breathing as you squat (as if you were sitting into a chair) through a count of 10 seconds. Hold for 2 seconds at the MTP. Push through your heels as you return to starting point through a count of 10 seconds. Without resting, repeat three times.

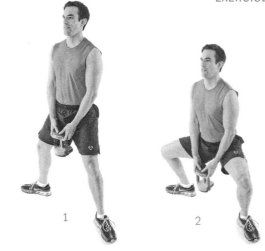

BACK

EXERCISE B

"W" Pull-down on Cable Machine

With the pulleys on their highest settings, grasp both handles with your palms facing each other. Sit back onto your heels, and keep your chest up and abs tight. Feather your breathing as you pull the weight down through a count of 10 seconds. Hold and squeeze for 2 seconds at the MTP (where your elbows touch your sides). Return the weight to starting point through a count of 10 seconds. Without resting, repeat three times.

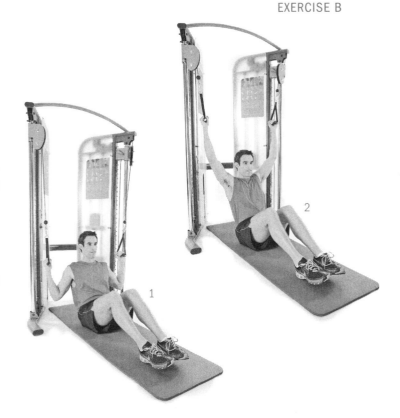

KEY: MTP: maximum tension point. **Feather your breathing:** Inhale deeply and exhale in short bursts.
Timing: Each exercise should take 90 seconds, and each circuit should take 6 minutes.

CHEST

EXERCISE C

Standard Push-up

Lie on a mat with your hands slightly
wider than shoulder-width apart and
your fingers pointing forward. Press up to
starting position, keeping your back
straight, abs tight, and head up. Feather
your breathing as you lower your chest
toward the floor through a count of
10 seconds. Hold for 2 seconds at the MTP.
Push your body back to starting position
through a count of 10 seconds, keeping
your elbows slightly bent. Without
resting, repeat three times.

ABS

EXERCISE D

Jackknife

Begin by standing about 3 feet in front
of the ball, and place the palms on the
ground, shoulder-width apart. From
here, put one foot on the ball about
mid-shin level. Then place the other foot
on the ball, keeping your head forward,
spine straight, and abs tight. Slowly pull
your knees up to your chin through a
count of 10 seconds, as you
concentrate on keeping stability by
squeezing your abs tight. Hold and
squeeze for 2 seconds at the MTP.
Return to starting point through a count
of 10 seconds. Without resting, repeat
three times.

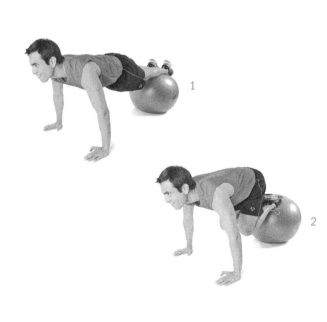

LEGS

Bench Squat on Cable Machine

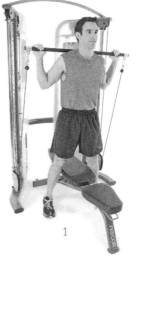
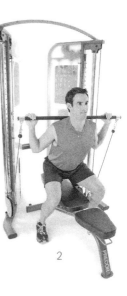

With the pulleys on their lowest settings, sit on the bench with the bar resting on your upper back, feet slightly wider than shoulder-width apart. Keep your back straight, abs tight, and head up. From here, stand to starting position. Feather your breathing as you squat (as if you were about to sit on the bench) through a count of 10 seconds. Hold for 2 seconds at the MTP, about 2 inches from touching the bench. Push through your heels as you stand up to starting position through a count of 10 seconds. Without resting, repeat three times. ***Backup move:*** *Plié Squat, page 66.*

BACK

Bent-over Row on Cable Machine (underhand grip)

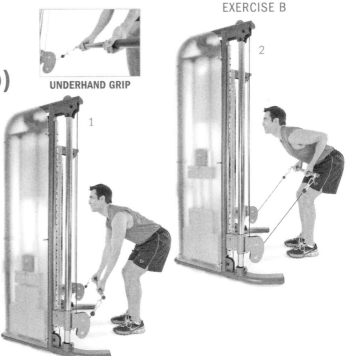

UNDERHAND GRIP

With the pulleys on their lowest settings, hold the bar using the underhand grip. Bend at the waist as if tying your shoes, and then lift only your chin and chest, creating a slight arch in the back while keeping a slight bend in your knees. Feather your breathing as you pull the bar up and back toward your hips through a count of 10 seconds, keeping your elbows close to the sides of your body. Hold and squeeze your shoulder blades together at the MTP for 2 seconds. Lower the bar back to starting position through a count of 10 seconds. Without resting, repeat three times. ***Backup move:*** *Bent-over Row (underhand grip), page 76.*

KEY: MTP: maximum tension point. **Feather your breathing:** Inhale deeply and exhale in short bursts.
Timing: Each exercise should take 90 seconds, and each circuit should take 6 minutes.

CHEST

Incline Cable Barbell Press on Swiss Ball

With the pulleys on their lowest settings, grip the bar about twice shoulder-width apart and lie on the ball so that your head and neck are supported. Allow your hips to drop almost to the ground. Extend your arms and feather your breathing as you lower the bar toward the top of your sternum through a count of 10 seconds. Hold for 2 seconds at the MTP. Press the bar up to starting point (just prior to lockout) through a count of 10 seconds. Without resting, repeat three times. **Backup move:** Incline Press on Swiss Ball, page 63.

EXERCISE C

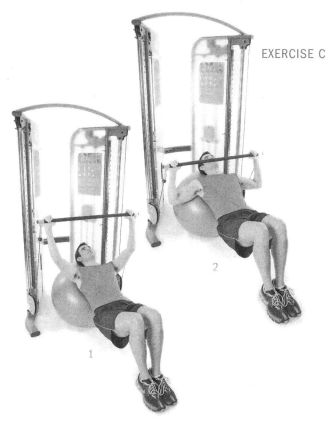

ABS

Cable Crunch on Knees

Grasp the rope attachment with the pulley on its highest setting. Hold the rope at the top of your head as shown. Kneel on your knees and avoid sitting back on your heels. Keeping your abs tight, feather your breathing as you bring your elbows toward your knees through a count of 10 seconds. Hold and squeeze for 2 seconds at the MTP. Return to starting point through a count of 10 seconds. Without resting, repeat three times.

EXERCISE D

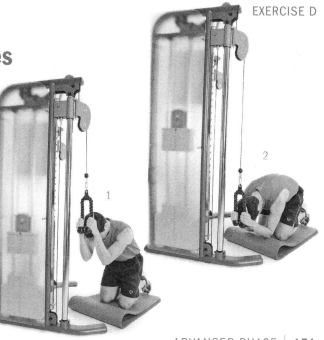

LEGS

EXERCISE A

Hamstring Kickback on Bench (cable optional)

With the pulley on its lowest setting, attach the cable to the ankle attachment. Place one knee on the bench, with both hands supporting your weight. Keep your head up and back straight throughout the exercise, with your foot flexed. Feather your breathing as you lift the other leg up and back through a count of 10 seconds, keeping your leg locked out and toes flexed. Hold and squeeze for 2 seconds at the MTP. Return to starting point through a count of 10 seconds. Without resting, repeat once more, then switch sides and complete 2 more reps, for a total of 4 reps. ***Backup move:*** *Glute Kickback on Swiss Ball, page 78.*

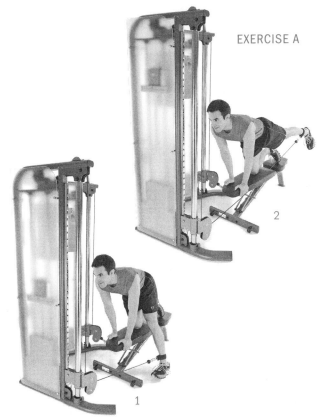

BACK

EXERCISE B

Hyperextension on Roman Chair

Position yourself on a Roman chair, with your arms crossed in front of you. Bend at the waist. Feather your breathing as you raise your upper body through a count of 10 seconds. Hold and squeeze for 2 seconds at the MTP. Lower to starting position through a count of 10 seconds. Without resting, repeat three times. (Note: The MTP will change depending on your level of flexibility.)

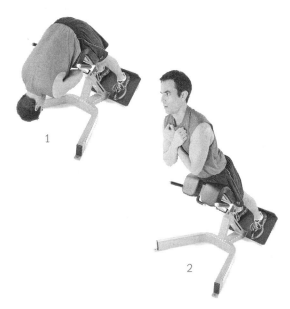

KEY: MTP: maximum tension point. **Feather your breathing:** Inhale deeply and exhale in short bursts.
Timing: Each exercise should take 90 seconds, and each circuit should take 6 minutes.

CHEST

Upward Cable Fly

EXERCISE C

Set the pulleys on their lowest settings. Grasp the handles with palms facing outward and take a lunge position. Feather your breathing as you raise the cables forward, squeezing them together throughout the movement. Hold and squeeze at the MTP for a count of 2 seconds. Resist the weight back to its starting position through a count of 10 seconds. Without resting, repeat three times. **Backup move:** *Incline Dumbbell Fly on Swiss Ball, page 77.*

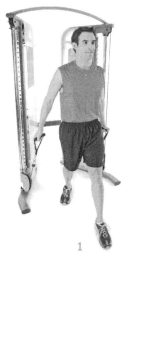
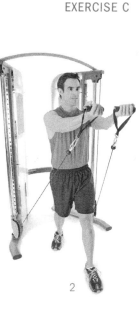

ABS

Cable Oblique Twist on Ball

EXERCISE D

Grasp the handle attachment, with the pulley about waist level. Lie on the ball with your head and neck supported, keeping your hips up, arms straight, and abs tight. Feather your breathing as you rotate your torso through a count of 10 seconds. Hold and squeeze for 2 seconds at the MTP (when your arms are parallel to the floor). Rotate back to starting point through a count of 10 seconds. Without resting, repeat three times. **Backup move:** *Russian Twist, page 85.*

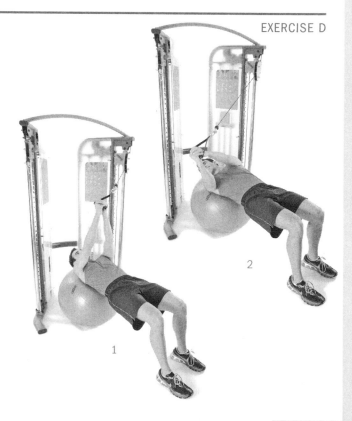

FINISH

SHOULDERS

EXERCISE A

Seated Shoulder Press on Bench

Hold a dumbbell in each hand as you sit on an upright bench. With your palms facing forward and extend the weights up over your head. Feather your breathing as you lower the weights down through a count of 10 seconds. Hold and squeeze for 2 seconds at the MTP (chin-level). Press the weight to starting point through a count of 10 seconds. Without resting, repeat three times.

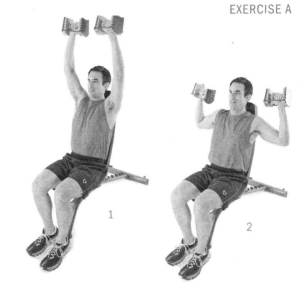

BICEPS

EXERCISE B

Reclined Cable Bar Curl

Grip the bar attachment with the pulleys on their lowest settings. Sit back into the incline bench, keeping your elbows by your sides, arms fully extended. Feather your breathing as you curl the bar up through a count of 10 seconds. Hold and squeeze at the MTP (where the biceps are fullly contracted) for 2 seconds. Lower the bar to starting point through a count of 10 seconds. Without resting, repeat three times. (Note: Keep your elbows tight against your body throughout the exercise.) **Backup move:** *Standing Curl, page 68.*

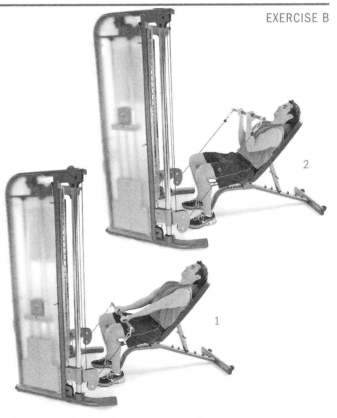

KEY: MTP: maximum tension point. **Feather your breathing:** Inhale deeply and exhale in short bursts.
Timing: Each exercise should take 90 seconds, and each circuit should take 6 minutes.

TRICEPS

EXERCISE C

Overhead Triceps Cable Extension

Set the pulleys on their lowest settings. Grip the bar attachment with your palms facing the ceiling, and sit on the incline bench with your chest up and abs tight. Extend your arms, keeping your biceps tight against your head. Feather your breathing as you lower the bar behind your head through a count of 10 seconds. Hold for 2 seconds at the MTP (when the elbow is at a 90-degree angle). Extend the bar to starting point through a count of 10 seconds. Without resting, repeat three times. (Note: Avoid letting your elbows drift outward or arching your back throughout this exercise.) **Backup move:** *Overhead Triceps Extension on Swiss Ball, page 81.*

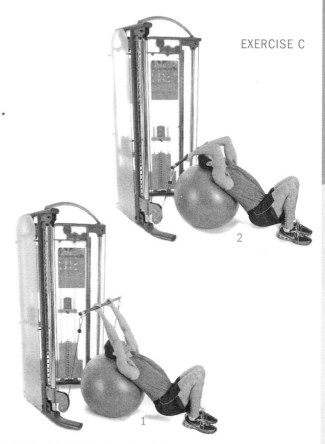

ABS

EXERCISE D

Jackknife

Standing about 3 feet in front of the ball, place the palms on the floor, shoulder-width apart. From here, put one foot on the ball about mid-shin level. Then place the other foot on the ball, keeping your head forward, spine straight, and abs tight. Slowly pull your knees up to your chin through a count of 10 seconds, as you concentrate on maintaining stability by squeezing your abs tight. Hold and squeeze for 2 seconds at the MTP. Return to starting point through a count of 10 seconds. Without resting, repeat three times.

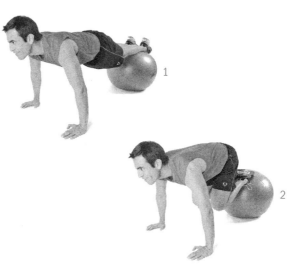

SHOULDERS

Standing Cable Lateral Raise

With the pulleys on their lowest settings, grasp the handles using the cross grip. Stand upright, keeping your abs tight and back straight. Feather your breathing as you raise the handles through a count of 10 seconds. Hold and squeeze for 2 seconds at the MTP. Then lower the weight to starting point through a count of 10 seconds. Without resting, repeat three times. **Backup move:** *Standing Lateral Raise, page 70.*

EXERCISE A

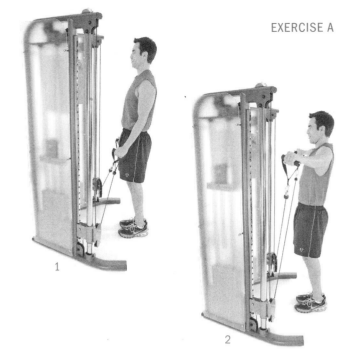

BICEPS

EXERCISE B

Incline Biceps Curl

Hold a pair of dumbbells and sit back into an incline bench, allowing your arms to hang down naturally, palms facing forward. Feather your breathing as you curl the dumbbells up through a count of 10 seconds. Hold and squeeze for 2 seconds at the MTP. Lower the weights to starting point through a count of 10 seconds, until your arms are completely straight at the bottom (do not lock your elbows). Without resting, repeat three times. (Note: Keep your elbows tight against your body throughout the exercise.)

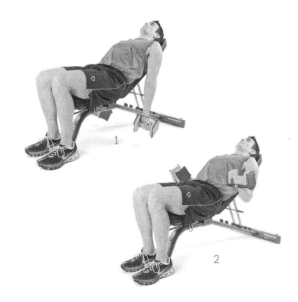

KEY: MTP: maximum tension point. **Feather your breathing:** Inhale deeply and exhale in short bursts.
Timing: Each exercise should take 90 seconds, and each circuit should take 6 minutes.

TRICEPS

EXERCISE C

Triceps Cable Press-down with Rope

Grasp the rope with the pulley on its highest setting, palms facing each other. Hold your elbows against your sides and lower the rope to about chest level. Feather your breathing as you pull the rope down through a count of 10 seconds, rotating your hands out at the end of the motion. Hold and squeeze at the MTP (just prior to lockout) for 2 seconds. Resist the weight back to starting point through a count of 10 seconds. Without resting, repeat three times. ***Backup move:*** *Chair Dip, page 69.*

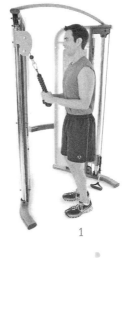

1

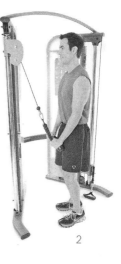

2

ABS

EXERCISE D

Standing Cable Crunch on Swiss Ball

Grasp the rope with the cable on the highest setting. Stand with the ball between you and the machine, supporting your lower back. Hold the rope to the back of your head as shown. Walk your feet in front of you about half a foot, with a slight bend in your knees. Feather your breathing as you curl your abs in and up, bringing your elbows toward your knees. Hold and squeeze for 2 seconds at the MTP. Return to starting point through a count of 10 seconds. Without resting, repeat three times.

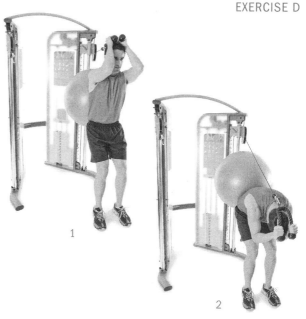

1

2

SHOULDERS

Recline Rear Delt Cable Extension

With the pulleys on their highest settings, grasp the handles using a cross grip and lie back into the inclined bench, with your arms extended and elbows slightly bent. Feather your breathing as you extend your arms back in an "arch" motion through a count of 10 seconds. Hold and squeeze for 2 seconds at the MTP. Return to starting point through a count of 10 seconds. Without resting, repeat three times. **Backup move:** *Bent-over Rear Delt Raise, page 98.*

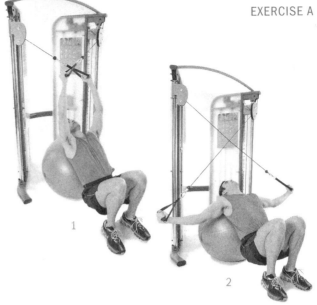

EXERCISE A

1

2

BICEPS

Cable Preacher Curl on Swiss Ball

Using the bar attachment with the pulleys on their lowest settings, lean over the ball with your knees on the floor and grab the bar, hands about 1 foot apart, palms facing up. Extend your elbows and feather your breathing as you curl the weight up through a count of 10 seconds. Hold and squeeze at the MTP for a count of 2 seconds. Lower the weight to starting point through a count of 10 seconds. Without resting, repeat three times. (Note: The preacher curl is the only curl in which you shouldn't allow your arms to extend fully. Keep your arms slightly bent at the bottom of the motion.) **Backup move:** *Preacher Curl on Swiss Ball, page 72.*

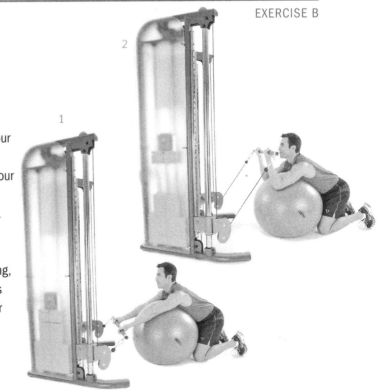

EXERCISE B

2

1

KEY: MTP: maximum tension point. **Feather your breathing:** Inhale deeply and exhale in short bursts. **Timing:** Each exercise should take 90 seconds, and each circuit should take 6 minutes.

TRICEPS

EXERCISE C

Close-Grip Cable Bench Press on Swiss Ball

With the pulleys on their lowest settings, lie on your back on the ball with your head and neck supported, keeping your hips up, arms straight, and abs tight. Grip the bar attachment with your hands about 6 inches apart and extend your arms in front of you. Feather your breathing as you lower the weight through a count of 10 seconds. Hold for 2 seconds at the MTP. Press the bar up to starting point through a count of 10 seconds. Without resting, repeat three times. **Backup move:** *Close-Grip Diamond Push-up on Knees, page 83.*

ABS

EXERCISE D

Wood Chopper

Grasp the handle or rope with the pulley on its highest setting and step about 2 feet away from the machine. Place your legs about 3 feet apart; keep your chest up, back and arms straight. Feather your breathing as you pull the cable down and across your body by twisting and contracting your obliques through a count of 10 seconds. Hold and squeeze for 2 seconds at the MTP. Resist the weight to starting point, through a count of 10 seconds. Without resting, repeat once more on this side and then switch sides and complete 2 more reps, for a total of 4. **Backup move:** *Broomstick Twist, page 67.*

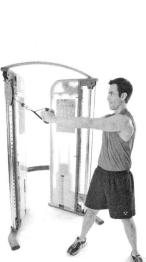

CONGRATULATIONS ON COMPLETING YOUR 8-WEEK CHALLENGE

AFTER THE 8-WEEK CHALLENGE

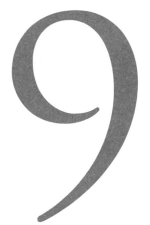

Doing the exercises helps me feel stronger in my daily life. **I plan to continue this program for the rest of my life!**

—BARBARA SEIDEL, *12-Second Star, lost 13 pounds*

If you are reading this chapter, you have most likely completed the 12-Second Sequence™ 8-Week Challenge. Yeah! Congratulations. I am so proud of you and all your hard work. You've made phenomenal progress over these last eight weeks, and I want you to feel great about your accomplishment. You deserve it.

Now that you've come this far, my challenge to you is to ***keep moving forward!*** We hope the last eight weeks inspired you to embrace this as a *lifestyle change,* not as something you do for a little while and then stop. When you continue beyond the 8-week Challenge, your results will also continue. The new muscle you put on your body is going to burn more and more calories while you're at rest.

One of the best rewards of your new healthy way of living may come when you go to the doctor. Many of my clients have talked about how their weight-loss and fitness improvements always get a big thumbs-up from their doctors. As you now know, losing weight now and—here's the key—*staying in shape* decreases such serious health risks as diabetes, heart disease, and certain forms of cancer. Think of the 12-Second Sequence™ as the ultimate insurance plan! Remember, your workout and nutrition knowledge are *good* habits to have in your life—like brushing your teeth. Good habits like these are going to ensure that you live a long, healthy, and happy life.

KEEP MOVING FORWARD

Now you've reached a new stage in your mental and physical development. When my oldest son stopped crawling and started walking, it was an important moment in his life, because it meant that he'd reached a more advanced state of development. Once he found a new and better way to move around, he didn't want to go back to crawling. *It's the same with your health and fitness.* Now that you've learned a new, healthier, more active way of living, you'll never go back to your old lifestyle. The rewards—a slimmer waistline, a better body, more confidence, more energy, and better all-around health—are just too great.

To stay on track with the 12-Second Sequence™, here are some key strategies to keep you moving forward with your success:

- Take pictures of where you are now to keep a visual record of your progress as you move into another 8-Week Challenge.
- Continue tracking your weight each week. Set a day every week to weigh yourself. I recommend Sunday, but it could be any day that falls after you've completed the two workouts. If you've been using the workout log system (from the resources section), keep recording your weight change there to hold yourself accountable. Remember that there's a space to record your inches, too—sometimes this can be a better indicator than the scale of the improvements in your body.
- Keep eating every three hours! When you advance to your next round of eight-week workouts, remember that sticking to your eating plan is key. As you continue to see improvements, you can make adjustments that suit your progress, but no matter what you do to monitor yourself, eating every three hours is critical to continue burning fat and building muscle.

LOSING MORE

I hope you've been using the workout logs and eating planner on pages 175–177 to record your experience. Keep these old logs and review them when you begin your next 8-Week Challenge to maximize your workouts and get the best results possible. Did you find that the Quick-Start Phase worked better for you because you liked being in the comfort of your own home? Or did you love being in the gym because it was more challenging and really accelerated your results? Learn from the past and you will ensure that your next 8-Week Challenge is even better. By the time you complete your third 8-Week Challenge, this new lifestyle will be automatic for you. *How should you start your next 8-Week Challenge exactly?* There are two options when it comes to keeping the 12-Second Sequence™ working for you:

1. **Stick with the Original Course.** As they say, if it ain't broke, don't fix it! If you liked the progression from dumbbells to the FT cable machine and felt that that provided the best buildup of a challenge for you, just stick with it.
2. **Mix It Up!** You can trade out different weeks to keep your ongoing fitness regimen exciting and fun. This means that you can do one week at home and another week in the gym or vice versa. Simply continue using the workout logs on pages 176 and 177 and customize new workout routines. For example, you might select the following for a Day 1 workout: a leg exercise from Week 5, a chest exercise from Week 6, a chest exercise from Week 1, and finally an ab exercise from Week 8. It's okay to mix it up. It's that simple. Check out 12second.com for our online library of exercises that you can personalize and mix up. *It's pretty cool!*

ADDITIONAL TIPS TO STAY FIT FOREVER

In chapter 5 we discussed creating a support team, whether that's a family member or a friend or a whole group of people. It's still important to maintain that support system! Your support team will help you stay motivated, challenge you to push yourself beyond your limits, and listen to you when you need to talk about your feelings. You may want to recruit a new workout partner or support buddy for your next 8-Week Challenge. You could even consider becoming a mentor—someone who is going to help change someone else's life. Think about how great you feel; is there someone in your life who could benefit from your experience with the 12-Second Sequence™? Tell them about the program and get them excited about seeing their best body ever!

The changes that you've made to your life can improve not just your life, but also the lives of your friends and family. As we discussed in chapter 1, over 60 percent of Americans are overweight or obese. This isn't just a matter of looks; when you're overweight, your quality of life suffers and your risk of developing life-threatening illnesses increases. When you take steps to make yourself healthier, as you have, you lengthen the time you have to spend with your loved ones. What's more, you improve the quality of that time. That's why it is so vital that you consider this a new way of life that you will continue for as long as you can. You, your friends, and your family will thank you for making the effort to live your best life possible.

As you continue with your progress, remember how important it is to track it. **And don't forget to join 12Second.com and post your before and after pictures as you keep up the amazing work.** I want to hear all about your results! You never know, I might call you personally to congratulate you. Regardless, congratulations on the new you, and I wish you all the best as you continue through this incredible journey.

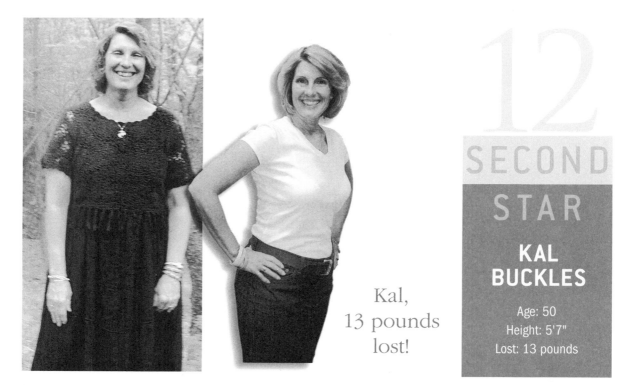

Kal,
13 pounds
lost!

12
SECOND
STAR

**KAL
BUCKLES**

Age: 50
Height: 5'7"
Lost: 13 pounds

"When I heard about the 12-Second Sequence™, I was approaching fifty and I had gained a lot of weight—menopause is no fun! I had bought every patch, pill, and exercise machine over the years to help me lose weight, and I finally just said, 'I'm done.' I wanted something simple and workable and something that gave me an option to take it with me wherever I go. The 12-Second Sequence™ gave me all of those things.

"The workouts were easy to follow and fit into my life. Before, I was working out six days a week, doing both cardio and strength training. But now, in just 20 minutes, twice a week, I see great results. I have a lot more energy and a lot more confidence. This program has made me feel like I can do anything I want to do—with fitness and with my life."

KAL'S SECRETS TO SUCCESS

· Drink the protein shakes—they keep you full!
· Form buddy groups.
· Cardio first thing in the morning—really gets you motivated to start your day.

FREQUENTLY ASKED QUESTIONS 10

What if I have *more time* and want to exercise daily?

This is a great question. I would not do more than the two resistance training sessions a week. You really must have the other days in the week off to let your muscles recuperate. But here is what I would recommend: ***power walking.*** I power-walk on a treadmill each morning. Although the program has cardio built in via the circuit training component, the human heart was designed to be pushed every day. What are the benefits of power walking? Well, it's perfect for boosting energy and getting an endorphin high. It's low-impact as well, so you won't stress your joints. It's a great way to maximize your energy first thing in the morning. Shoot for an intensity level of about 7 to 8 on a scale of 1 to 10. The key to achieving this intensity is adding an incline to your walk. If you can, find an area in your neighborhood or at a nearby park that has some nice hills to walk. This will help get your heart rate going quickly and boost the benefits of your morning cardio. If you plan on doing the walk indoors on a treadmill, the same rule applies—add to the incline until you feel your breathing getting just beyond a comfortable conversation level. That will ensure it's a "power" walk.

Now, as I mentioned in chapter 6, here is a little secret: Do it first thing in the morning *on an empty stomach*. Research done at Kansas State University has shown that you'll burn more calories if you do cardio before breakfast than if you eat first. And one other study, conducted at the University of California, Berkeley, confirmed this by finding that fat loss increased *only* when the study participants "exercised in a fasted state." Your body fasts at night when you are sleeping, and your metabolism naturally slows down because your body needs less energy. So when you get your energizing power walk in first thing in the morning, you rev your metabolism from the very start of your day.

How much more will you burn if you power walk on an empty stomach? Well, if you keep it to 20 minutes, which is the ideal, you will burn a bonus 150 to 200 calories a day. So let's say you walk before breakfast six times a week. That's up to *1,200 more calories a week* you could be burning. It definitely is not as effective as the 12-Second Sequence's™ power to burn fat and reshape your body, but it is a really nice bonus.

What if it takes me too long to transition between moves at the gym?

Once you begin Week 5 and you start working out in the gym you may notice that it's tougher to transition directly into your next move—don't get discouraged! Remember to review the day's workout before you begin so you're already familiar with the sequence of moves—and then just do your best to keep your transition time to a minimum. It's important to keep moving so that your heart rate stays up and you receive the benefits of the circuit-training element, but a few seconds will not undo the effects of your 12-Second Sequence™ workouts. If you're in a real crunch, refer to the backup moves to help you maintain your pace.

What if I don't feel the burn?

If you're counting correctly throughout your 10-second motions and 2-second holds, you should feel a significant burn when you finish each set. If you aren't feeling that burn, your form or your intensity may not be ideal. To get the most out of your workout, make sure that you maintain proper form. This means that you feel the stress of each move on the muscle you're working. Don't let surrounding muscles support your movements. When you do a biceps curl, for example, you should feel the full weight of the dumbbell or cable on your biceps, not your back or shoulders. Bad form not only cheats you of an effective workout, but also puts you at risk for debilitating injuries.

Intensity is just as important to getting maximum results as form. Since you're only doing four reps per exercise, it's important to make those reps count. This workout is only 20 minutes, twice a week, so giving it your best is crucial. The most critical element regarding intensity is choosing the right weight. You should pick a weight that completely fatigues the muscle after four reps. If you can do only two or three reps, the weight is too heavy. If you can do five or six reps, the weight is too light. Remember, you can only create new lean muscle tissue if you completely fatigue muscles, and correct form and intensity are essential to your success.

What if I don't want to go to the gym?

For the absolute best results, you should take advantage of the last four weeks of the program in the gym. There is simply no true replacement for the way a functional trainer will challenge your muscles. However, if it's impossible for you to make it to the gym, you can repeat the first four weeks of the 12-Second Sequence™ for a total of eight weeks. This is not an ideal alternative, but you will absolutely see amazing results. But, I recommend you follow the program as it's designed. Once you become acquainted with your local gym, I guarantee you'll be thrilled with the trimmed and tone results you'll see in the mirror!

Do I really have to avoid eating starchy carbs at night?

Yes!! Following this part of the eating plan is absolutely critical to your success. After your afternoon snack, you must commit to avoiding carbs high in starch. Most of us are less active in the evening than we are during the day, so our bodies don't require as much energy. Starchy carbs are designed to give you high energy, so if you *don't* use them, they'll be stored as fat. Read more about nonstarchy carbs and other ideal food sources in chapter 4.

I feel like I'm eating too much food! Do I have to eat everything on my plate?

The last thing I want you to do is overeat! My first suggestion is to eat until you're satisfied and comfortable. Remember, if you weigh under 150 pounds, eat 3 ounces of protein at each meal; if you weigh over 150 pounds, eat 5 ounces. It's important to get the ideal amount of protein, so try your best to stick to the guidelines. If you eat the recommended amounts of protein, carbs, and fat, you should feel satisfied and not overly full.

Is there an alternative to the whey protein shake for my snack?

Whey protein is the most bioavailable source of protein, which means that it's the easiest source for your body to digest. This is why protein shakes are your ideal snacks on the 12-Second Sequence™. Like we discussed earlier, whey protein shakes are the best way to feed your muscles what they need to build and repair themselves after your workouts. I understand that you might want some other option, however. So the next best option is low-fat (2 percent) cottage cheese. A half cup is only 100 calories, has only 2 grams of fat, and provides over 15 grams of good protein. But remember, you are here to create your best-looking body ever . . . you need to keep it simple and effective. See the resources section for other alternatives to whey protein shakes.

Can I replace my meals with whey protein shakes?

No. I recommend that you eat normal meals for breakfast, lunch, and dinner. I would not replace any of your three main meals with a whey shake; keep them for your snacks exclusively. But, if you do need a quick breakfast that you can take with you on-the-go, look for my Protein-Packed Breakfast Smoothie recipe on page 182. It's quick, easy, delicious, and you can take it with you when you're in a rush!

Should I continue with an exercise if I experience pain?

First, you should know that there are two types of pain: "good" pain and "bad" pain. When you work out with the 12-Second Sequence™ and you truly challenge your muscles, you will experience the good kind. When you feel the burn as you count through your last ten seconds of an exercise move, you're creating the resistance that will transform your lean muscle tissue. You may feel a bit sore after some of the exercises—and that's great because it means that you're challenging your muscles. The bad kind of pain is an injury or an aggravation of a pre-existing injury. If this is the pain you feel, **stop immediately.** If you ignore it and continue to exercise or "push through it," you will probably cause more damage. If you have a preexisting injury or health condition, I recommend seeing your physician before starting the 12-Second Sequence™ or any other exercise program.

Will the 12-Second Sequence™ make me look big and bulky?

There are two parts to this answer. If you are a woman, then the answer is no, absolutely not. Women lack the high amount of testosterone necessary to create big and bulky muscles, and can only create big muscles with the use of steroids. The second part to this answer is for men. Guys, you *can* get big with the 12-Second Sequence™. You will add muscle mass because the testosterone levels in the male body allow for that kind of development, but you'll discover that the exercises give you defined, toned muscles, not blocky, shapeless ones.

Do I need to stretch before starting my workout?

It's true that if you don't stretch before, during, and after performing an exercise, you can very likely cause an injury. One of the unique aspects of the 12-Second Sequence™, though, is that it has a built-in warm-up element. Because the exercises are done at such a slow pace and the weight, if you're using one, is much lighter than what you would normally lift, you actually stretch your muscles as you perform the moves. You also won't be doing any quick, explosive movements that would shock resting muscles. Stretching is great for you, though, so don't be afraid to stretch out your muscles on the days you're not working out.

How can I overcome a plateau?

If you hit a plateau, the first thing you should do is go back and take a look at your "before" picture. This will show you how far you have come since you started, and will give you a fresh perspective on your progress. Another thing to do is take a week off. This may sound like the last thing you'd expect to hear, but taking a short break can help you regroup and gather your motivation. You may also need an environment change. Try shifting the location of your workouts. For the first four weeks, you could even try doing them outside, since you only need a few materials. I also strongly suggest you review the eating plan and make sure you're getting in your protein shakes and keeping the starchy carbs out of your evening diet—staying disciplined with these two elements of the eating plan can make all the difference.

I need *extra motivation*. Jorge, can you coach me personally?

YES! The best way to visit me is online at 12second.com. And when you become a club member, I will coach you daily through streaming video sessions; I'll be there with you every day of your 8-Week Challenge. It's important to have a coach, and I look forward to having you join me online as my client.

Do you have a video of the 12-Second Sequence™?

Yes, I have two great DVD kits that you can get at 12second.com or anywhere fitness videos are sold, or you can download them at iTunes.com. One is a simple Intro Kit that offers the first full week of exercises, which will be a great jump-start to get you going. The other is the complete Quick-Start Phase. This features the first two weeks of the 12-Second Sequence™. Either way, it's like having me personally coach you in your living room! Check 12second.com for availability.

Where can I get more planners and logs?

Since our program is a 56-day plan, you will really need to stay organized with *both* the exercise and the eating. This is why I created an 8-week companion journal that you can find on our website or wherever books are sold. It has great daily inspirational quotes and logs for all your workouts and eating. There is also a digital option available when you visit 12second.com: You can download and print a 7-Day Grid that will track your eating *and* your workouts. Even better, when you join 12second.com, you can print a customized grid with *your workouts and meals already filled in!* I've done all the work for you.

Where can I send my before and after pictures?

You can post your before and after photos with your story on our 12Second.com site. I might select you to be in a future 12-Second Sequence™ book, on the website, or on a national television show with me.

I have more questions. Where can I ask them?

Visit our 12second.com site, where you can access my "Ask Jorge" database, which has even more frequently asked questions. See you there!

COLLIN STRICKLAND

Age: 22
Height: 5'7"
Lost: 12 pounds

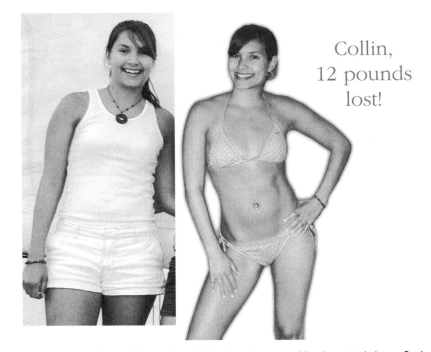

Collin, 12 pounds lost!

"I just graduated from college where I drank and ate anything I wanted. Jorge Cruise taught me what it means to make healthy choices and how to stick with them. I actually get excited to do my workouts, knowing what a difference they make not only on my appearance, but also with my self-esteem. My body is leaner and more toned; I feel like a different person when I put on my 'skinny' jeans—the ones I had shoved in the back of my closet. My relationship with food has completely changed. Unlike other diets, Jorge Cruise explains how your body reacts to certain foods. I am so lucky to have experienced this program at twenty-two because I feel healthy and motivated to make the new me last forever."

COLLIN'S SECRETS FOR SUCCESS

· Don't give up. Each day write out what you eat and how you feel about the food and/or workout.
· Lay out your workout clothes the night before—cuts time in the morning and lessens the chances of you skipping your morning cardio.
· Keep snacks around you so you never miss snack time.

RESOURCES

The Workout Logs and Eating Planner on the following pages will help keep you organized during your 8-Week Challenge. Photocopy these charts, three-hole–punch them, and place them in a binder. You'll need eight copies of each Workout Log and fifty-six copies of the Eating Planner. Or you can get a copy of the *12-Second Sequence™ Journal,* which has these logs as well as inspirational quotes and meditations. You can also visit 12second.com to download and print a 7-Day Grid in order to log your eating and your workouts on one sheet. Choose a method that works for you so you stay motivated and organized throughout your challenge.

DATE: _____

EATING PLANNER

This plan will ensure leaner muscle and a higher metabolism.

Breakfast>time _____   Description

○ **PROTEIN*** (3-5oz/40g)	
○ **CARBS** (½ cup or 1 slice of bread)	
○ **FRUIT** (1 cup)	
○ **FAT** (1 teaspoon)	

Snack>time _____   Description

○ **WHEY PROTEIN SHAKE** (1 scoop)	

Jorge recommends Jorge's Packs™ for your protein drinks. > See list of other recommended snacks on page 204.

Lunch>time _____   Description

○ **PROTEIN*** (3-5oz/40g)	
○ **CARBS** (½ cup or 1 slice of bread)	
○ **VEGGIES**** (2 cups)	
○ **FAT** (1 teaspoon)	

Snack>time _____   Description

○ **WHEY PROTEIN SHAKE** (1 scoop)	

Dinner>time _____   Description

○ **PROTEIN*** (3-5oz/40g)	
○ **VEGGIES**** (2-4 cups)	
○ **FAT** (1 teaspoon)	

Snack>time _____   Description

○ **WHEY PROTEIN SHAKE** (1 scoop)	

*If you weigh less than 150 pounds, eat 3 ounces of protein at every meal; if you weigh more than 150 pounds, eat 5 ounces of protein.

**Veggies = nonstarchy vegetables.

Water (eight 8-oz cups)   ○ ○ ○ ○ ○ ○ ○ ○

Multivitamin   ○

Primary Workout

DATE_____ DAY_____ OF 56

Start>time_____ Finish>time_____

TOTAL TIME_____

Select weights so that by the end of the 4th rep of each exercise you feel an intensity level of 8.

CIRCUIT 1

Muscle Group	Exercise	Weight Used	Intensity Level
LEGS			
BACK			
CHEST			
ABS			

At this point you should be about 6 minutes into your workout.

CIRCUIT 2

Muscle Group	Exercise	Weight Used	Intensity Level
LEGS			
BACK			
CHEST			
ABS			

At this point you should be about 14 minutes into your workout, including 2 minutes of transition time.

CIRCUIT 3

Muscle Group	Exercise	Weight Used	Intensity Level
LEGS			
BACK			
CHEST			
ABS			

At this point in your workout you should be at 20 minutes. Congratulations! YOU DID IT!

BONUS CARDIO 26-MINUTE MORNING POWER WALK ○

After my workout I feel _____

(e.g., confident, strong)

Secondary Workout

DATE_____ DAY_____ OF 56

Start>time_____ Finish>time_____

TOTAL TIME_____

Select weights so that by the end of the 4th rep of each exercise you feel an intensity level of 8.

CIRCUIT 1

Muscle Group	Exercise	Weight Used	Intensity Level
SHOULDERS			
BICEPS			
TRICEPS			
ABS			

At this point you should be about 6 minutes into your workout.

CIRCUIT 2

Muscle Group	Exercise	Weight Used	Intensity Level
SHOULDERS			
BICEPS			
TRICEPS			
ABS			

At this point you should be about 14 minutes into your workout, including 2 minutes of transition time.

CIRCUIT 3

Muscle Group	Exercise	Weight Used	Intensity Level
SHOULDERS			
BICEPS			
TRICEPS			
ABS			

At this point in your workout you should be at 20 minutes. Congratulations! YOU DID IT!

BONUS CARDIO 26-MINUTE MORNING POWER WALK ◯

After my workout I feel_____

(e.g., confident, strong)

8-WEEK WORKOUT CHART

Start>date _____   Finish>date _____

	Monday	Tuesday	Wednesday	Thursday	Friday	Saturday	Sunday	
	DAY 1 PRIMARY WORKOUT	**DAY 2** DAY OFF	**DAY 3** DAY OFF	**DAY 4** SECONDARY WORKOUT	**DAY 5** DAY OFF	**DAY 6** DAY OFF	**DAY 7** DAY OFF	WEEK 1
	DAY 8 PRIMARY WORKOUT	**DAY 9** DAY OFF	**DAY 10** DAY OFF	**DAY 11** SECONDARY WORKOUT	**DAY 12** DAY OFF	**DAY 13** DAY OFF	**DAY 14** DAY OFF	WEEK 2
	DAY 15 PRIMARY WORKOUT	**DAY 16** DAY OFF	**DAY 17** DAY OFF	**DAY 18** SECONDARY WORKOUT	**DAY 19** DAY OFF	**DAY 20** DAY OFF	**DAY 21** DAY OFF	WEEK 3
	DAY 22 PRIMARY WORKOUT	**DAY 23** DAY OFF	**DAY 24** DAY OFF	**DAY 25** SECONDARY WORKOUT	**DAY 26** DAY OFF	**DAY 27** DAY OFF	**DAY 28** DAY OFF	WEEK 4
	DAY 29 PRIMARY WORKOUT	**DAY 30** DAY OFF	**DAY 31** DAY OFF	**DAY 32** SECONDARY WORKOUT	**DAY 33** DAY OFF	**DAY 34** DAY OFF	**DAY 35** DAY OFF	WEEK 5
	DAY 36 PRIMARY WORKOUT	**DAY 37** DAY OFF	**DAY 38** DAY OFF	**DAY 39** SECONDARY WORKOUT	**DAY 40** DAY OFF	**DAY 41** DAY OFF	**DAY 42** DAY OFF	WEEK 6
	DAY 43 PRIMARY WORKOUT	**DAY 44** DAY OFF	**DAY 45** DAY OFF	**DAY 46** SECONDARY WORKOUT	**DAY 47** DAY OFF	**DAY 48** DAY OFF	**DAY 49** DAY OFF	WEEK 7
	DAY 50 PRIMARY WORKOUT	**DAY 51** DAY OFF	**DAY 52** DAY OFF	**DAY 53** SECONDARY WORKOUT	**DAY 54** DAY OFF	**DAY 55** DAY OFF	**DAY 56** SUCCESS!	WEEK 8

*Please photocopy and place on your refrigerator. As you complete your workouts, cross off the days so you can see your success!

7-DAY MENU PLANNER

This is a sample planner. The amount of protein you eat will vary based on your weight. Please see page 32 for guidelines.

Day 1
Breakfast:	**Protein Oatmeal**
Snack:	1 whey protein shake (Jorge's Packs™)
Lunch:	**Spicy Chipotle Salmon**
Snack:	1 whey protein shake (Jorge's Packs™)
Dinner:	**Mediterranean Chicken**
Snack:	1 whey protein shake (Jorge's Packs™)

Day 2
Breakfast:	**Protein-Packed Breakfast Smoothie**
Snack:	1 whey protein shake (Jorge's Packs™)
Lunch:	**Green Chile Cheeseburger**
Snack:	1 whey protein shake (Jorge's Packs™)
Dinner:	**Portobello Pizza**
Snack:	1 whey protein shake (Jorge's Packs™)

Day 3

Breakfast:	**Fruit and Cottage Cheese Parfait**
Snack:	1 whey protein shake (Jorge's Packs™)
Lunch:	**Ginger Lime Grilled Shrimp Salad**
Snack:	1 whey protein shake (Jorge's Packs™)
Dinner:	**Spaghetti with Meat Sauce**
Snack:	1 whey protein shake (Jorge's Packs™)

Day 4

Breakfast:	**Mushroom Spinach Breakfast Burritos**
Snack:	1 whey protein shake (Jorge's Packs™)
Lunch:	**Curried Chicken Salad in Lettuce Cups**
Snack:	1 whey protein shake (Jorge's Packs™)
Dinner:	**Asian Pork Tenderloin with Bok Choy**
Snack:	1 whey protein shake (Jorge's Packs™)

Day 5

Breakfast:	**Steak and Eggs with Potato Hash**
Snack:	1 whey protein shake (Jorge's Packs™)
Lunch:	**White Bean and Tuna Sandwiches**
Snack:	1 whey protein shake (Jorge's Packs™)
Dinner:	**Grilled Halibut with Romesco Sauce**
Snack:	1 whey protein shake (Jorge's Packs™)

Day 6

Breakfast:	**Spicy Southwestern Frittata**
Snack:	1 whey protein shake (Jorge's Packs™)
Lunch:	**Greek Chicken Pita Pockets**
Snack:	1 whey protein shake (Jorge's Packs™)
Dinner:	**Filet Mignon with Cabernet Sauce**
Snack:	1 whey protein shake (Jorge's Packs™)

Day 7   FREE DAY!

12-SECOND SEQUENCE™ RECIPES

These recipes were formulated with 5 ounces of protein per serving. Adjust the amount of protein to suit your needs based on your weight. Remember, if you weigh less than 150 pounds, eat 3 ounces of protein per serving. If you weigh more than 150 pounds, eat 5 ounces. Visit 12second.com for more recipe ideas.

Breakfast
Protein Oatmeal
Protein-Packed Breakfast Smoothie
Fruit and Cottage Cheese Parfait
Steak and Eggs with Potato Hash
Smoked Salmon Scramble
Spicy Southwestern Frittata
Mushroom Spinach Breakfast Burritos

Lunch
Spicy Chipotle Salmon
Green Chile Cheeseburgers
Ginger Lime Grilled Shrimp Salad
White Bean and Tuna Sandwiches
Shrimp and Black Bean Tostadas
Greek Chicken Pita Pockets
Curried Chicken Salad in Lettuce Cups

Dinner
Mediterranean Chicken
Portobello Pizza
Spaghetti with Meat Sauce
Grilled Halibut with Romesco Sauce
Spinach-Stuffed Chicken Breasts
Filet Mignon with Cabernet Sauce
Asian Pork Tenderloin with Bok Choy

Bonus Recipe
Lemon Flax Vinaigrette

Protein Oatmeal

Warm, comforting oatmeal is a delicious and healthy way to start your day. Oatmeal provides high-quality fiber, protein, and numerous vitamins and minerals, such as vitamin E, zinc, selenium, iron, and magnesium. Oatmeal has even been shown to help reduce the risk of developing heart disease and several types of cancers.

Serves 4
Cooking time: 15 minutes

1 teaspoon kosher salt

2 cups rolled oats

3 scoops Jorge's Packs™ whey protein powder

4 cups blueberries

4 teaspoons flaxseed oil

In a medium saucepan over medium heat, bring $3\frac{1}{2}$ cups water to a boil and add salt. Stir in the oats and protein powder and bring back to a boil. Reduce heat to low and simmer, uncovered, stirring occasionally, until the oatmeal is tender, 10 to 15 minutes. Remove from heat and stir in the blueberries and flaxseed oil. Divide among four bowls and serve.

Protein-Packed Breakfast Smoothie

This smoothie is a sweet, delicious, nutritious, and easy way to start your morning. Vary your fruits so that your smoothie is refreshing and different every day.

Serves 1
Prep time: 5 minutes

$\frac{1}{2}$ medium ripe banana

1 cup frozen fruit (mango, raspberries, blueberries, cherries, pineapple, peaches)

$\frac{1}{2}$ cup unsweetened apple juice

$\frac{1}{2}$ cup vanilla soy milk

1 teaspoon flaxseed oil

1 scoop Jorge's Packs™ vanilla whey or other protein powder

Combine all ingredients in a blender and puree until smooth. Serve.

Fruit and Cottage Cheese Parfait

Cottage cheese is an ideal choice for your meals on the 12-Second Sequence™. Not only is it low in fat and calories, but it also provides plenty of high-quality protein.

In a medium bowl, combine the cottage cheese and the Forti-Flax. Place ¼ cup cottage cheese in the bottom of each of four tall clear parfait glasses. Top with ¼ cup raspberries. Continue layering cheese and berries and top the parfait with the last of the berries. Toast bread and spread with fruit spread. Serve each person one parfait and one slice of toast.

Serves 4
Prep time: 5 minutes

4 cups low-fat cottage cheese

4 tablespoons Barlean's Forti-Flax

4 cups raspberries

4 slices whole grain bread

4 teaspoons all-fruit spread

Steak and Eggs with Potato Hash

This dish is a perfect breakfast for meat lovers. Precooked diced potato makes this dish quick and easy, while beef tenderloin and fried eggs fill you up. Enjoy this diner favorite and know that you're treating your body well.

Serves 4

Cooking time: 15 minutes

2 teaspoons olive oil

2 cups precooked diced potatoes

Salt and pepper

½ onion, diced

1 green bell pepper, diced

2 tablespoons chopped flat-leaf parsley

Cooking spray

Four 4-ounce 95 percent lean beef tenderloin fillets, trimmed of all visible fat

4 large eggs

4 medium oranges

Heat a large nonstick skillet over medium-high heat and add the oil. Add the potatoes to the skillet and season with salt and pepper. Sauté until potatoes begin to brown, about 5 minutes. Add the onion and bell pepper and stir to combine. Continue to sauté until onion and pepper soften and brown, about 5 minutes more. Reduce heat to low, taste for seasoning, and stir in parsley.

Meanwhile, heat another large nonstick skillet over high heat and spray with cooking spray. Season steaks with salt and pepper and add to skillet. Sear the steaks to desired doneness, about 3 minutes per side for medium rare. Remove from skillet and tent with foil to keep warm.

Lower the heat under the skillet to medium and spray with cooking spray. Carefully break the eggs into the skillet. Fry eggs until the whites look mostly set, then flip. Fry for 10 seconds more and remove from heat.

Divide the hash among four plates. Top the hash with one egg and add one steak to each plate. Serve with oranges.

Smoked Salmon Scramble

Smoked salmon with cream cheese is a natural flavor pairing. Combined with scrambled eggs and fresh dill, this scramble makes a delicious breakfast any day of the week. Toast and sweet cantaloupe round out this mouth-watering meal.

Heat a large nonstick skillet over medium heat and spray with cooking spray. Lightly beat the eggs and egg whites in a large bowl. Add eggs to the skillet and scramble, stirring lightly until they look about half cooked. Stir in salmon, diced cream cheese, and dill. Continue cooking, lightly stirring, until semisoft curds form. Season to taste with salt and pepper.

Toast bread and spread with fruit spread. Serve each person one fourth of the salmon scramble, one slice of toast, and 1 cup of cantaloupe cubes.

Serves 4
Cooking time: 10 minutes

Cooking spray

6 eggs

8 egg whites

4 ounces smoked salmon, cut into strips

2 tablespoons reduced-fat cream cheese, diced

2 tablespoons chopped fresh dill

Salt and pepper

4 slices whole grain bread

4 teaspoons all-fruit spread

4 cups cantaloupe cubes

Spicy Southwestern Frittata

Serves 4
Cooking time: 15 minutes

6 eggs

12 egg whites

2 scallions, sliced

2 tablespoons chopped cilantro

Salt and freshly ground black pepper

Cooking spray

1 garlic clove, minced

½ chipotle chile, canned in adobo sauce, minced

½ cup canned black beans, rinsed and drained

½ cup prepared salsa

2 soft taco-size Mission® 98 percent fat-free tortillas

4 medium apples

Ever been to New Mexico? This frittata will get you close! All the classic Southwestern flavors—cilantro, beans, smoked chiles, and garlic—combine to make this frittata a homespun version of the American Southwest. Beware of the chipotles in adobo—they pack a seriously spicy punch!

Preheat broiler.

In a large bowl, whisk together the eggs, egg whites, scallions, and cilantro, and season with salt and pepper.

Heat a large nonstick skillet over medium heat and spray with cooking spray. Add garlic and chipotle, and sauté until garlic is fragrant, 1 minute. Add black beans and stir to combine. Add egg mixture to skillet and gently stir to combine. Cook eggs until edges start to set, 3 to 4 minutes. Place under broiler to finish cooking, 4 to 5 minutes.

Cut frittata into four wedges. Serve each person one wedge topped with salsa, half of a tortilla, and one apple.

Mushroom Spinach Breakfast Burritos

Mushrooms and spinach create a delicious flavor combination in these light, tasty burritos. Two cups might seem like a lot of spinach, but it cooks down to almost nothing in the heat of the pan.

Heat a large nonstick skillet over medium heat and spray with cooking spray. Add mushrooms and sauté until golden, 5 to 6 minutes, and season to taste with salt and pepper. Add spinach and sauté until wilted.

Lightly beat the eggs and egg whites in a large bowl. Add eggs to the pan. Cook until bottom begins to set, stirring to scramble. Stir in diced bell pepper. Taste for seasoning and adjust if necessary.

While the eggs cook, heat tortillas in microwave, 30 seconds. Divide egg mixture evenly among the tortillas. Roll into a burrito shape and serve each person one burrito and one orange.

Serves 4
Cooking time: 10 minutes

Cooking spray

1 cup sliced mushrooms

Salt and freshly ground black pepper

2 cups fresh baby spinach

6 eggs

12 egg whites

1 roasted bell pepper, diced

4 soft taco-size Mission® 98 percent fat-free tortillas

4 small oranges

Spicy Chipotle Salmon in Foil Packets

Cooking fish in foil is a quick and easy way to infuse the fish with rich flavor and keep it tender and moist. In this recipe, luscious salmon is topped with a sweet and spicy chipotle butter. The butter melts into a unique, complex sauce that delicately coats the salmon. Paired with a fresh green salad, this spicy salmon will become a staple at your dinner table.

Serves 4
Cooking time: 15 minutes

4 teaspoons unsalted butter, softened

1 chipotle chile, canned in adobo sauce, minced

1 tablespoon adobo sauce

½ teaspoon kosher salt

¼ teaspoon freshly ground black pepper

½ teaspoon brown sugar, packed

Four 6-ounce salmon fillets

2 tablespoons chopped fresh cilantro

12 cups mixed salad greens

1 cup sliced mushrooms

3 scallions, sliced

1 cup cherry tomatoes, halved

2 cups fat-free croutons

½ cup fat-free ranch dressing

Lime wedges

Preheat oven to 400°F.

Combine the butter, chipotle, adobo, salt, pepper, and sugar in a small bowl. Stir until well combined.

Tear off four sheets of aluminum foil, each about 1 foot long. Place one piece of fish in the center of each piece of foil and season with salt and pepper. Spread each piece of fish with 1 teaspoon of the chipotle butter and sprinkle with ½ tablespoon cilantro. Fold the foil over itself and scrunch the ends together to seal.

Place the packets on a sheet pan and bake 8 to 10 minutes until fish flakes easily with a fork.

Toss the greens, mushrooms, scallions, tomatoes, croutons, and dressing in a large bowl. Divide among four salad plates.

Serve each person one fish packet with lime wedges and one salad.

Green Chile Cheeseburgers

Canned green chiles come in hot and mild varieties. If you're sensitive to spicy foods, you can still enjoy these cheeseburgers and reap the benefits of chile peppers. Chiles have been used to treat asthma, arthritis, blood clots, and headaches, among other conditions. Some people even claim that chiles aid weight loss! So pile them on—they're good for you!

Place the ground turkey in a large bowl and add the Worcestershire, salt, and pepper. Combine gently, taking care not to overwork the meat (overmixing will make your burgers tough). Form the turkey into four patties and place in the fridge to rest while you prepare the remaining ingredients.

Heat a grill or grill pan over medium heat. Place the patties on the grill and cook, turning once, until browned on the outside and cooked throughout, about 4 to 5 minutes per side. Don't press down on the burgers with a spatula as they cook; you'll just squeeze all the moisture out of them. Toward the end of the cooking process, top each burger with one slice of cheese and continue grilling until cheese melts.

While the burgers grill, heat the green chiles in a small saucepan over medium heat. Place one cheeseburger on each bun half. Top each with one fourth of the green chile, one onion slice, one tomato slice, ¼ cup spinach, and one bun top.

Toss salad greens with dressing in a large bowl. Divide among four salad plates.

Serve each person one burger and one salad.

Serves 4
Cooking time: 15 minutes

1¼ pound ground turkey

1 tablespoon Worcestershire sauce

1 teaspoon kosher salt

1 teaspoon freshly ground black pepper

Two 1-ounce slices reduced-fat cheddar, halved

Two 4-ounce cans hot or mild green chiles, drained

4 whole-grain hamburger buns, halved

4 thin slices red onion

4 large slices tomato

1 cup baby spinach

8 cups mixed salad greens

½ cup fat-free salad dressing

Ginger Lime Grilled Shrimp Salad

Serves 4
Cooking time: 10 minutes

1½ pounds large uncooked shrimp, peeled and deveined

2 tablespoons plus ½ teaspoon minced fresh ginger

Zest of 2 limes

4 garlic cloves, minced

1 teaspoon kosher salt

1 teaspoon freshly ground black pepper

Cooking spray

Juice of 2 limes

1 tablespoon soy sauce

1 teaspoon honey

1 teaspoon sesame oil

1 tablespoon extra virgin olive oil

4 ounces rice noodles

2 cups thinly sliced Napa cabbage

2 red bell peppers, thinly sliced

3 scallions, sliced

2 tablespoons chopped mint

2 tablespoons chopped cilantro

4 cups mixed baby greens

2 tablespoons peanuts, toasted and chopped

If you like Thai food, but don't like the heat of its characteristic chiles, then this dish is for you. This refreshing salad combines elements of Thai cuisine, such as ginger, lime, and soy sauce, but doesn't contain anything spicy. This meal makes great leftovers, too, because the shrimp are delicious hot or cold. Just make sure you toss the salad with the dressing right before you eat it, not the night before.

Combine the shrimp, 2 tablespoons ginger, lime zest, 3 garlic cloves, salt, and pepper in a large zip-top bag. Massage ingredients in bag until shrimp are well coated in the marinade. Refrigerate for 8 hours or overnight. Let shrimp sit out at room temperature for about 20 minutes before cooking.

Heat a grill or grill pan over medium-high heat and spray with cooking spray.

In a small bowl, whisk together the lime juice, soy sauce, honey, sesame oil, remaining ginger and garlic, and olive oil. Adjust seasoning if necessary. Set aside.

Cook rice noodles according to package instructions. Toss with 2 tablespoons of the dressing and set aside.

Add shrimp to grill and cook, turning once, until opaque, about 2 minutes per side.

While the shrimp cook, combine the cabbage, bell peppers, scallions, mint, cilantro, and greens in a large bowl with remaining dressing. Toss to coat.

Divide salad evenly among four plates. Top each salad with one fourth of the vermicelli. Decoratively arrange the shrimp on each plate and sprinkle with peanuts. Serve.

White Bean and Tuna Sandwiches

This fresh, Mediterranean-style tuna salad replaces the fattening mayonnaise of traditional tuna salad with heart-healthy olive oil and fresh lemon juice. White beans add fiber, which helps you feel more full. This satisfying sandwich travels well, too—wrap up the pitas in foil and take them with you on the go!

In a medium bowl, combine the beans, tuna, onion, celery, capers, lemon zest and juice, olive oil, dill, and salt and pepper to taste. Fold ingredients together gently so you don't crush the beans.

Line each pita half with spinach and tomatoes. Stuff each pocket with one fourth of the tuna mixture. Serve each person one pita pocket half.

Serves 4
Prep time: 10 minutes

2 cups canned white beans (navy or cannellini), rinsed and drained

Two 6-ounce cans water-packed solid white albacore tuna

¼ red onion, diced

1 rib celery, diced

2 tablespoons capers

Zest and juice of 1 lemon

2 tablespoons extra virgin olive oil

1 tablespoon chopped dill

Salt and freshly ground black pepper

2 whole wheat pita pocket breads, halved

1 cup baby spinach leaves

2 tomatoes, sliced

Shrimp and Black Bean Tostadas

Tostadas are like tacos, but the shell is flat and the fillings are piled on top. Protein-rich shrimp and black beans fill this tostada that's topped with fresh veggies and light sour cream. Experiment with other fillings until you come up with your favorite combination.

Serves 4
Cooking time: 5 minutes

4 tostada shells

2 cups canned black beans, rinsed and drained

2 ounces reduced-fat cheddar cheese, shredded

1½ pounds medium shrimp, peeled and deveined

Salt and freshly ground black pepper

1 cup prepared green salsa

4 tomatoes, seeded and diced

2 green onions, sliced

4 cups baby spinach, roughly chopped

¼ cup chopped fresh cilantro

4 tablespoons low-fat sour cream

Preheat broiler. Line a baking sheet with foil and arrange tostada shells on the sheet. Evenly divide beans among tostada shells and sprinkle with cheese. Top with shrimp and season with salt and pepper. Broil tostadas until shrimp are opaque and cheese is melted, 2 to 3 minutes.

Remove tostadas from heat and top with salsa, tomatoes, onions, spinach, cilantro, and a tablespoon of sour cream. Serve each person one tostada.

Greek Chicken Pita Pockets

This sandwich is so quick and easy to throw together, you won't believe how delicious it is. Lean chicken breast is combined with cucumber, tomatoes, salty feta cheese, and briny olives to create a unique salad that's stuffed inside pita pockets. Wrap these sandwiches in foil to make a convenient, portable picnic lunch.

In a large bowl, combine chicken, spinach, cucumber, onion, tomatoes, feta, and olives. Season with salt and pepper and add vinaigrette. Toss to coat. Divide salad among pita halves. Serve each person one half sandwich.

Serves 4
Prep time: 10 minutes

1¼ pounds cooked chicken breast meat

2 cups baby spinach

¼ seedless cucumber, thinly sliced

¼ red onion, thinly sliced

1 cup cherry tomatoes, halved

2 ounces feta cheese, crumbled

6 kalamata olives, pitted and quartered lengthwise

Salt and freshly ground black pepper

½ cup reduced-fat red wine vinaigrette

2 whole wheat pita pocket breads, halved

Curried Chicken Salad in Lettuce Cups

Serves 4
Cooking time: 10 minutes

¾ cup quick-cooking brown rice

¼ cup reduced-fat mayonnaise

¼ cup plain low-fat yogurt

¼ cup chopped chives

¼ red onion, finely diced

1 rib celery, finely diced

Juice of 1 lime

1 tablespoon curry powder, or more to taste

1¼ pounds cooked chicken breast meat

2 tablespoons golden raisins

2 tablespoons slivered almonds, toasted

Salt and freshly ground black pepper

8 large cup-shaped Bibb or butter lettuce leaves

Our twist on chicken salad includes sweet golden raisins, spicy curry powder, and crunchy almonds. We've cut most of the fat from traditional chicken salad by using reduced-fat mayonnaise and yogurt instead of sour cream. Freshly chopped chives add a beautiful green accent to this yellow-hued salad. Serving this salad in lettuce cups makes it pretty enough for company.

Combine rice with 1½ cups water in a medium saucepan over medium-high heat. Bring to a boil and reduce heat to low. Simmer until the rice is tender and the water has been absorbed, about 10 minutes.

Meanwhile, stir together the mayonnaise, yogurt, chives, onion, celery, lime juice, and curry powder. Gently fold in chicken, raisins, and almonds. Season with salt and pepper.

Stack two lettuce leaves on each of four plates. Mound one fourth of the chicken salad into each lettuce cup. Add ½ cup of rice to each plate and serve.

Mediterranean Chicken

Mediterranean diets are rich in healthy fats (like olive oil), lean meats, and robust flavors. This recipe for Mediterranean Chicken brings the best of this Old World region to your dinner table in a matter of minutes. Smoky, grilled chicken breasts are topped with a zesty relish of kalamata olives and sun-dried tomatoes. Mediterranean Chicken is a delightful way to tour Europe from the comfort of your own dining table.

Heat a grill or grill pan over medium heat and spray with cooking spray. Season chicken with salt and pepper. Grill chicken until cooked through, 5 to 6 minutes per side.

While the chicken cooks, stir together the olives, tomatoes, capers, lemon zest, parsley, and olive oil in a small bowl.

In a large bowl, toss the spinach, greens, peppers, broccoli, and tomatoes with the vinaigrette. Divide among four salad plates.

Place one chicken breast on each of four plates. Top with one fourth of the olive-tomato mixture and 1 tablespoon feta cheese. Serve each person one chicken breast and one salad.

Serves 4
Cooking time: 15 minutes

Cooking spray

Four 6-ounce skinless chicken breast halves

Salt and freshly ground black pepper

½ cup kalamata olives, pitted and quartered lengthwise

½ cup sun-dried tomatoes (not oil-packed), chopped

2 tablespoons capers, rinsed and drained

½ teaspoon grated lemon zest

2 tablespoons chopped flat-leaf parsley

1 tablespoon extra virgin olive oil or flaxseed oil

6 cups baby spinach

6 cups mixed baby greens

2 red bell peppers, sliced

2 cups broccoli florets

1 cup cherry tomatoes, halved

½ cup fat-free vinaigrette

¼ cup crumbled feta cheese

Portobello Pizza

Serves 4
Cooking time: 20 minutes

Cooking spray

4 large portobello mushroom caps

Salt and freshly ground black pepper

1 cup prepared marinara sauce

10 ounces cooked chicken breast meat, shredded

2 ounces part-skim mozzarella, grated

2 ounces Parmesan cheese, grated

¼ cup chopped flat-leaf parsley

8 cups green beans, trimmed

Just because you've adopted a healthier new lifestyle doesn't mean that some of your favorite foods, like pizza, are off limits. Our unique twist on pizza uses a delicious, meaty portobello mushroom as the crust and tops it with lean chicken breast and low-fat cheese. Experiment with this technique to create your own healthy pizza recipes.

Heat a grill or grill pan over medium-high heat and spray with cooking spray. Preheat broiler. Bring a large pot of salted water to a boil and add a steamer basket.

With a small spoon, scrape out the brown gills on the inside of the mushroom caps and discard. Season the mushrooms with salt and pepper and add to the grill. Grill until the mushrooms are tender, turning occasionally, 4 to 5 minutes. Remove mushroom caps from the grill and place on a sheet pan.

While the mushrooms grill, heat the marinara sauce in a small saucepan over medium heat.

Top each mushroom with ¼ cup marinara sauce. Divide the chicken evenly among the four caps. Sprinkle with mozzarella and Parmesan. Place under the broiler until cheese melts and browns, 3 to 4 minutes, rotating the pan occasionally. Remove from broiler and sprinkle with parsley.

Meanwhile, when the water comes to a boil, add the green beans and cover. Steam until tender, 6 to 8 minutes. Drain and season with salt and pepper.

Serve each person one pizza with 2 cups of green beans.

Spaghetti with Meat Sauce

The 12-Second Sequence™ omits carbs in the evening, but you can still enjoy a traditional pasta dish. Spaghetti squash is a tasty, low-calorie winter squash with long strands of flesh that resemble strands of pasta. Topped with a savory meat sauce, our version of this classic is so delicious, you'll never miss the empty carbs!

Serves 4
Cooking time: 15 minutes

1 tablespoon olive oil

¾ pound ground turkey

¾ pound ground turkey breast

Salt and pepper

½ onion, finely diced

4 garlic cloves, minced

1 cup finely diced mushrooms, about 6 large

2 cups prepared marinara sauce

¼ cup chopped flat-leaf parsley

1 large spaghetti squash

12 cups mixed salad greens

½ cup fat-free vinaigrette

¼ cup grated Parmesan

Heat the oil in a large, straight-sided sauté pan over medium heat. Add the ground turkey and turkey breast, season with salt and pepper, and cook until browned. Add the onion, garlic, and mushrooms and sauté until the vegetables are tender and the mushrooms have given off most of their liquid, 5 minutes. Add the sauce and parsley and adjust the seasoning if necessary. Simmer for 10 minutes.

Meanwhile, cut the squash in half lengthwise and remove the seeds. Place cut side up in a microwave-safe baking dish and season with salt and pepper. Pour ⅓ cup water into the dish and microwave on high for 10 to 15 minutes or until tender. Remove from microwave and cool. Pat dry with paper towels.

While the squash cools, toss the salad greens with the vinaigrette in a large bowl. Divide among four salad plates.

When the squash is cool enough to handle, use a fork to scrape the long strands of flesh from the shells. Divide the squash among four pasta bowls, 1 cup per serving. Top the squash with one fourth of the meat sauce. Sprinkle each bowl with 1 tablespoon grated Parmesan.

Serve each person one bowl of squash and one salad.

Grilled Halibut with Romesco Sauce

Romesco sauce, a classic from the Catalonia region of Spain, combines roasted peppers, tomatoes, onions, garlic, almonds, and olive oil. In this recipe, we've paired this flavorful sauce with meaty grilled halibut. Garnished with bright green parsley, this meal looks as good as it tastes.

Serves 4
Cooking time: 15 minutes

Cooking spray

Four 6-ounce halibut steaks

Salt and freshly ground black pepper

4 roasted red bell peppers (you can use the kind that come in a jar, but drain them)

2 cups canned fire-roasted tomatoes, drained

¼ red onion, coarsely chopped

2 tablespoons slivered almonds, toasted

2 garlic cloves

2 tablespoons sherry vinegar

2 tablespoons extra virgin olive oil

8 cups mixed salad greens

½ cup sliced red onions

½ cucumber, sliced

½ cup sliced mushrooms

½ cup low-fat vinaigrette

¼ cup chopped flat-leaf parsley

Heat a grill or grill pan over medium-high heat and spray with cooking spray.

Season fish with salt and pepper and place on the grill. Grill halibut steaks until they flake easily with a fork, about 5 minutes per side.

While the fish grills, combine the peppers, tomatoes, chopped onion, almonds, garlic, vinegar, salt, and pepper to taste in a food processor or blender. Pulse the sauce, streaming the olive oil until well combined. Taste for seasoning and set aside.

In a large bowl, toss the salad greens with the sliced onions, cucumber, mushrooms, and vinaigrette, and divide among four salad bowls.

Serve each person one salad and one halibut steak topped with one fourth of the romesco sauce. Garnish with parsley.

Spinach-Stuffed Chicken Breasts

Part-skim ricotta, vitamin-rich spinach, and fresh basil make a creamy, delectable filling for protein-packed lean chicken breasts. Paired with lemon-almond steamed broccoli, this meal tastes as luscious as it looks.

Preheat oven to 425°F.

Heat a small skillet over medium heat and add olive oil. Add onion and garlic. Sweat vegetables until soft and translucent. Remove from heat and set aside to cool.

In a small bowl, stir together the spinach, ricotta, salt and pepper to taste, basil, and cooled onion mixture until well combined. Place mixture in a large zip-top bag. Squeeze the mixture down to one corner of the bag and snip off the tip.

Holding each chicken breast lengthwise, make a small incision through the side of the thicker end with a sharp, narrow knife (like a boning knife). With the tip of the knife pointing toward the small end of the breast, carefully edge the knife back and forth to create a pocket inside the breast. Take care not to slice the breast open. Repeat with remaining breasts.

Season the breasts inside and out with salt and pepper. Place the cut end of the bag holding the filling inside the chicken pockets. Squeeze about one fourth of the filling into each chicken breast. Secure the open ends with toothpicks. Spread the tops of the chicken breasts with 1 tablespoon mustard.

Spray a sheet pan with cooking spray. Place the stuffed chicken breasts on the sheet pan and bake until they reach an internal temperature of 165°F, 15 to 20 minutes.

While the chicken bakes, bring 2 inches of water to a simmer in a large stockpot and add a steamer basket. Add the broccoli and cover. Steam broccoli until tender, 6 to 8 minutes. Remove from heat and toss with almonds and lemon zest and juice. Season with salt and pepper.

Serve each person one stuffed chicken breast and 1½ cups broccoli.

Serves 4
Cooking time: 20 minutes

1 tablespoon olive oil

½ medium onion, finely diced

2 garlic cloves, minced

One 10-ounce package frozen chopped spinach, thawed and squeezed dry

1 cup part-skim ricotta

Salt and freshly ground black pepper

2 tablespoons chopped basil

Four 6-ounce boneless, skinless chicken breast halves

4 tablespoons Dijon mustard

Cooking spray

6 cups broccoli florets

2 tablespoons sliced almonds, toasted

Zest and juice of 1 lemon

Filet Mignon with Cabernet Sauce

This meal rivals a steak dinner at your favorite steakhouse. Keep in mind that the flavor of the wine intensifies as it reduces in the sauce, so choose a wine that you would enjoy from a glass.

Serves 4
Cooking time: 15 minutes

Four 5-ounce 95 percent lean beef tenderloin fillets, trimmed of all visible fat

Salt and pepper

Cooking spray

1 large shallot, diced

2 garlic cloves, chopped

2 sprigs thyme

1 cup cabernet sauvignon (or other red wine)

1 cup low-sodium beef broth

2 heads cauliflower, chopped

1 tablespoon unsalted butter

2 tablespoons skim milk

2 pounds asparagus, trimmed

Bring a large pot of salted water to a boil. Heat a large sauté pan over medium-high heat.

Season the steaks with salt and pepper. Add steaks to the sauté pan and sear to desired doneness, 3 minutes per side for medium rare. Remove steaks and place on a plate tented with foil to keep warm.

Spray the pan with cooking spray and add the shallot, garlic, and thyme, and sauté until vegetables are tender. Deglaze the pan with the wine and broth, scraping the pan with a wooden spoon to loosen any browned bits from the bottom. Bring the liquid to a boil and reduce by half, 5 minutes. Taste for seasoning and adjust if necessary.

While the sauce reduces, add the cauliflower to the boiling water and cook until tender. Strain the cauliflower, leaving the water in the pot, and add to a food processor. Add the butter and milk and process until smooth. Season to taste with salt and pepper.

Bring the water back to a boil, add the asparagus, and cook until tender, 3 to 4 minutes. Drain asparagus and season with salt and pepper.

Serve each person one filet mignon topped with one fourth of the cabernet sauce, $\frac{1}{2}$ cup of the pureed cauliflower, and one fourth of the asparagus.

Asian Pork Tenderloin with Bok Choy

This delicious marinade penetrates the pork to create a rich, intense Asian flavor. The reduced marinade makes a perfect light dressing for the smoky, grilled bok choy. The marinade is delicious with chicken as well as pork.

Serves 4
Cooking time: 15 minutes

1½ pounds pork tenderloin, trimmed of all visible fat

¼ cup soy sauce

2 tablespoons rice wine vinegar

1 tablespoon chile garlic sauce

2 teaspoons sesame oil

1 tablespoon hoisin sauce

1 tablespoon Worcestershire sauce

1 teaspoon chile oil

½ tablespoon oyster sauce

2 scallions, sliced

1 tablespoon chopped fresh ginger

3 garlic cloves, chopped

¼ cup chopped cilantro

½ teaspoon kosher salt

½ teaspoon freshly ground black pepper

Cooking spray

4 heads bok choy, halved lengthwise, roots kept intact

In a large zip-top bag, combine the pork, soy sauce, vinegar, chile garlic sauce, sesame oil, hoisin sauce, Worcestershire sauce, chile oil, oyster sauce, scallions, ginger, garlic, cilantro, salt, and pepper. Massage the bag to coat the pork in the marinade. Marinate the pork for 8 hours or overnight, massaging the bag occasionally to distribute the marinade.

Heat grill or grill pan over medium-high heat and spray with cooking spray. Remove the pork from the marinade and pat dry with paper towels. Reserve the marinade. Grill the pork until the internal temperature reads 145°F. Remove from heat and tent with foil to keep warm.

Pour the marinade into a small saucepan over high heat. Bring mixture to a boil and reduce by half. Set aside.

Spray the bok choy with cooking spray and season with salt and pepper. Grill the bok choy until the stems are tender and the leaves are slightly charred, 2 minutes per side.

Slice the pork into ½-inch-thick slices. Divide the pork among four dinner plates. Add two bok choy halves to each plate and drizzle with reduced marinade. Serve.

Lemon Flax Vinaigrette

I premiered this vinaigrette on *Emeril Live!* on the Food Network. You will love it!

¼ cup freshly squeezed lemon juice

1 garlic clove, mashed

1 teaspoon Dijon mustard

Pinch of salt

4 to 5 grinds black pepper

¼ cup flaxseed oil

¼ cup extra-virgin olive oil

Combine all ingredients in a jar with a tight-fitting lid. Shake to emulsify dressing. Taste for seasoning and serve.

IDEAL FOODS LIST

Here's a list of the best foods to choose when you're creating your own 12-Second Sequence™ meals. Be sure to stick to the recommended serving size for each meal to ensure your success.

Protein (3 ounces if you weigh less than 150 pounds; 5 ounces if you weigh more than 150 pounds)

- 95 percent lean beef
- Beef tenderloin
- Chicken/turkey breast (skinless)
- Eggs (whole)
- Fish
- Lamb
- London broil
- Low-fat cottage cheese
- Ostrich
- Pork tenderloin
- Round steak
- Shellfish

Carbohydrate (½ cup or 1 slice of bread)

- Brown rice
- Buckwheat
- Oatmeal
- Sweet potatoes
- Wheat germ
- Whole grain cereal
- Whole grain flour
- Whole wheat bread
- Whole wheat pasta
- Whole wheat tortilla
- Wild rice

Vegetables (Nonstarchy) (2 to 4 cups)

- Alfalfa sprouts
- Asparagus
- Beets (minimize)
- Bell peppers
- Broccoli
- Brussels sprouts
- Cabbage
- Cauliflower
- Celery
- Chiles
- Cucumber
- Eggplant (minimize)

- Garlic
- Green beans
- Green onions
- Lettuce
- Mushrooms
- Parsnips (minimize)
- Radishes

- Spinach
- Squash
- Tomatoes
- Turnips (minimize)
- Watercress
- Zucchini

Fats [1 teaspoon]

- Almonds (6)
- Almond butter
- Avocado ($\frac{1}{8}$)
- Cashews (6)

- Flaxseed oil
- Olive oil
- Peanut butter
- Peanuts (10)

Fruits [1 item or 1 cup diced]

- Apples
- Blackberries
- Blueberries
- Grapefruit
- Grapes
- Lemon

- Lime
- Melon
- Peaches
- Pears
- Strawberries

Snacks [3 per day]

- Jorge's Packs™ whey protein shake
- 6 ounces plain nonfat yogurt
- Low-fat cottage cheese ($\frac{1}{2}$ cup)

- 1 ounce beef jerky
- $\frac{1}{2}$ cup chopped cooked chicken breast
- 3 ounces tuna or salmon (canned or pouch)

Freebies

- Club soda
- Coffee (minimize)
- Diet soda (minimize)

- Mineral water
- Propel® Fit Water™
- Water

Sugar Substitutes [in moderation]

- Splenda®

- Stevia

Sweets [in moderation]

- Sugar-free candies
- Sugar-free gelatin desserts

- Sugar-free gum

Flavor Enhancers

- Garlic
- Herbs (fresh or dried)
- Lemon or lime juice
- Low-sodium broth
- Low-sodium soy sauce
- Mustard
- Pickles
- Salsa
- Spices
- Vinegar
- Worcestershire sauce

Supplements (use daily)

- Barlean's flaxseed oil
- Jorge's Packs™ Vitamins
- Jorge's Packs™ whey protein

FAST/FROZEN FOODS LIST

I am very busy, so I understand that sometimes you need to pick up something to eat on the go. Here are some of your best choices that you'll find at stores and restaurants in your area.

BREAKFAST

Fast Food

- Subway® Western Egg with Cheese Breakfast Sandwich (1)
  Add a piece of fruit.

- McDonald's® Egg McMuffin® (1)
  Add a piece of fruit.

- Denny's® Veggie Cheese Omelet with Egg Beaters® (1)
  Add a piece of fruit.

Frozen Food

- Weight Watchers® Smart Ones® English Muffin Sandwich (1)
  Add a whey protein shake and a piece of fruit.

- Lean Pockets® Bacon, Egg, and Cheese (1)
  Add a whey protein shake and a piece of fruit.

- Lean Pockets® Sausage, Egg, and Cheese (1)
  Add a whey protein shake and a piece of fruit.

LUNCH

Fast Food

· Arby's® Santa Fe Salad with Grilled Chicken (1)
Add one serving of light buttermilk ranch dressing.

· Baja Fresh® Shrimp Tacos (2)
Add a side salad (2 cups) and a squeeze of lemon for dressing.

· Blimpie® Turkey Sub, 6-inch, on whole wheat (1)

· Burger King® TenderGrill® Chicken Filet Salad (1)
Add one serving of Ken's® Fat-Free Ranch Dressing.

· Chick-fil-A® Chicken Cool Wrap® (1)
Add a side salad (2 cups) and a squeeze of lemon for dressing.

· Chick-fil-A® Southwest Chargrilled Chicken Salad (1)
Add a squeeze of lemon for dressing, half a packet of Garlic and Butter Croutons, and a small order of Hearty Breast of Chicken Soup.

· Chipotle Bol with Barbacoa (1)
Ask for double lettuce, fajita vegetables, red tomatillo salsa, and black beans. No rice.

· Dairy Queen® Grilled Chicken Sandwich (1)
Add a side salad with one serving of fat-free Italian dressing.

· KFC® Tender Roast® Sandwich without sauce (1)
Ask for an additional 2 ounces of grilled chicken and add a house side salad with Hidden Valley® Golden Italian Light Ranch Dressing.

· McDonald's® Asian Salad with Grilled Chicken
Ask for an additional 1 ounce of chicken and a side of Butter Garlic Croutons. Add a squeeze of lemon for dressing.

· Rubio's Fresh Mexican Grill® Mahi Mahi Taco (1)
Ask for an additional 3 ounces of mahi mahi and add side salad (2 cups) with 2 tablespoons salsa for dressing.

· Rubio's Fresh Mexican Grill® Carne Asada Street Tacos (2)
Ask for an additional 2 ounces of carne asada and add a half side order of pinto beans and a side salad (2 cups) with 2 tablespoons salsa as dressing.

- Rubio's Fresh Mexican Grill® HealthMex® Chicken Taco (2)
  Ask for an additional 1 ounce of chicken and add a side salad (2 cups) with 2 tablespoons salsa as dressing.

- Subway® Club Sandwich, 6-inch, on whole wheat (1)
  Add a Veggie Delite salad with fat-free Italian dressing.

Frozen Food

- Healthy Choice® Flavor Adventures Chicken Tuscany (1)
  Add a mixed green salad (2 cups) with a squeeze of lemon and 1 teaspoon flaxseed oil for dressing.

- Healthy Choice® Flavor Adventures Grilled Whiskey Steak (1)
  Add a mixed green salad (2 cups) with a squeeze of lemon and 1 teaspoon flaxseed oil for dressing.

- Lean Cuisine® Café Classics Chicken a L'Orange (1)
  Add a mixed green salad (2 cups) with a squeeze of lemon and 1 teaspoon flaxseed oil for dressing.

- Lean Cuisine® Casual Eating Classics™ Roasted Garlic Chicken Pizza (1)
  Add a mixed green salad (2 cups) with a squeeze of lemon and 1 teaspoon flaxseed oil for dressing.

- Lean Cuisine® One Dish Favorites™ Classic Five Cheese Lasagna (1)
  Add a mixed green salad (2 cups) with a squeeze of lemon and 1 teaspoon flaxseed oil for dressing.

DINNER

Fast Food

- Chipotle Bol with Chicken (1)
  Ask for double lettuce, fajita vegetables, green tomatillo salsa, and tomato salsa. No rice or beans.

- Daphne's® Greek Chicken Salad (1)
  Ask for no pita and extra salad. Add a squeeze of lemon for dressing.

- KFC® Roasted Caesar Salad (1)
  Ask for an additional 3 ounces of roasted chicken and Hidden Valley® Light Golden Ranch Dressing.

- McDonald's® Bacon Ranch Salad with Grilled Chicken (1)
  Ask for an additional 2 ounces of grilled chicken and Newman's Own® Low-Fat Balsamic Vinaigrette.

- Subway® Grilled Chicken Breast and Spinach Salad (1)
  Ask for an additional 3 ounces of grilled chicken and fat-free Italian dressing.

Frozen Food

- Gorton's® Cajun Blackened Grilled Fillets (3)
  Add mixed green salad (3 cups) with lemon juice and 1 teaspoon flaxseed oil for dressing.

- Gorton's® Shrimp Temptations Scampi (2 servings)
  Add mixed green salad (3 cups) with lemon juice and 1 teaspoon flaxseed oil for dressing.

- Tyson® Mesquite Breast Fillets (Bagged) (2)
  Add mixed green salad (3 cups) with lemon juice and 1 teaspoon flaxseed oil for dressing.

Note: For suggestions on dining in restaurants, whether Mexican, Italian, or Chinese, see chapter 4, page 36. And go to 12second.com for more fast/frozen foods ideas.

BONUS: WEIGHT-FREE ROUTINE

This on-the-go, customized workout is specifically designed for those times when you don't have access to a gym or workout equipment. This 12-exercise routine is formulated to work your whole body in just one 20-minute workout. You won't need a gym or any equipment. You only use your own body weight for resistance. This routine is perfect for when you're traveling or even when you're in your office at work! And, if you want me in your ear, coaching you through these workouts, be sure to pick up *The 12-Second Sequence*™ Audiobook. I'll take you through an audio training session of this weight-free routine. You can find it at any bookstore or at iTunes.

Lunge

Kneel down on one knee with about a 2-foot gap between your heel and knee. Stand up to starting position with your back straight, chest up, and abs tight. Feather your breathing as you drop your back knee toward the ground through a count of 10 seconds. Hold for 2 seconds at the MTP, about 1 inch above the ground. Return to starting position through a count of 10 seconds. Repeat one more time on this leg. Without resting, perform 2 more reps on the other side, for a total of 4 reps. (Note: To avoid injury, make sure that your front knee doesn't travel past your toes.)

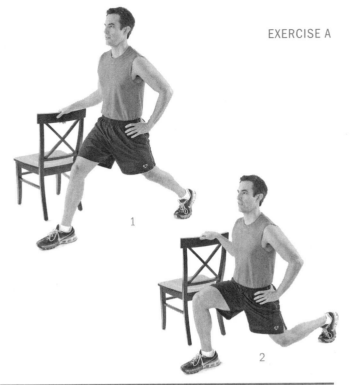

Push-up on Knees

Kneel on a mat on all fours with your knees hip-width apart. Your hands should be slightly wider than shoulder-width apart and your fingers pointing forward. Feather your breathing as you lower your chest toward the floor through a count of 10 seconds. Hold for 2 seconds at the MTP. Push your body back to starting position, keeping your elbows slightly bent, through a count of 10 seconds. Without resting, repeat three more times.

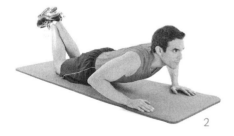

Chair Dip

Sit on the front edge of a chair with your hands close by your sides and fingers forward. With your legs extended, flex your feet so that your weight is on your heels. Feather your breathing as you slide away from the chair and lower yourself down through a count of 10 seconds. At the MTP, hold for 2 seconds. Lift yourself back up to starting point through a count of 10 seconds. Without resting, repeat three more times. (Note: Your MTP will depend on how flexible your shoulders are. Your MTP will be about an inch above your most flexible point.)

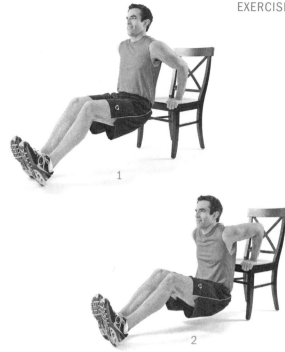

Toe Reach

Lie on your back. Cross your legs, flex your feet, and raise your legs up to 90 degrees. With your arms extended and chin up, feather your breathing as you crunch up and reach for your toes for a count of 10 seconds. Hold for 2 seconds at the MTP. Lower yourself back to starting position, keeping your shoulder blades from touching the ground, through a count of 10 seconds. Without resting, repeat three more times.

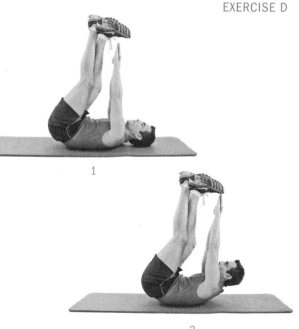

Beginner Squat

Stand between two sturdy chairs with your feet shoulder-width apart. Feather your breathing as you slowly squat through a count of 10 seconds, keeping your back straight, abs tight, and chest up. Hold for 2 seconds at the MTP. Return to starting position through a count of 10 seconds. Without resting, repeat three times. (Note: Be sure to use the chairs only for balance, not to hold your weight.)

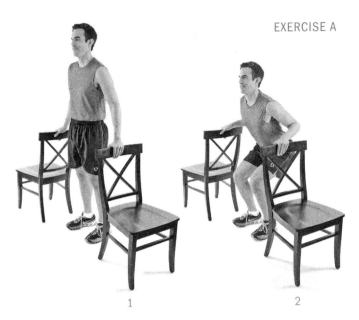

1

2

Bird Dog

Kneel on all fours with your knees hip-width apart. Keep your head up and abs tight throughout the exercise. Feather your breathing as you simultaneously lift and extend your left arm and your right leg through a count of 10 seconds. Hold and squeeze for 2 seconds at the MTP (when your arm and thigh are parallel to the floor). Return to starting position through a count of 10 seconds. Without resting repeat once more, then switch sides and complete 2 more reps for a total of 4 reps.

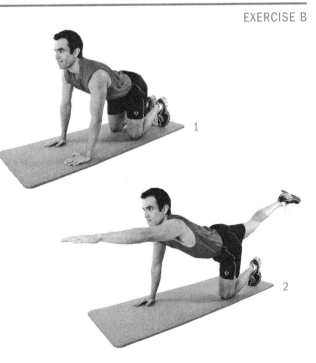

1

2

Diamond Push-up

EXERCISE C

Lie flat on a mat or towel. Extend your arms in front of you using the diamond position, and cross your ankles as you balance on your knees. Keeping your back straight and abs tight, feather your breathing as you lower your body down through a count of 10 seconds, allowing your elbows to move outward. Hold for 2 seconds at the MTP, about 2 inches above the ground. Return to starting position through a count of 10 seconds. Without resting, repeat three more times.

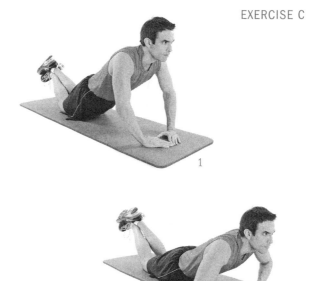

Reverse Crunch

EXERCISE D

Lie flat on a mat with your hands by your sides, palms down. Pull your heels up as close to your butt as possible. Raise your heels up about 2 inches off the ground. Keep your chin up and abs tight. Feather your breathing as you pull your knees up using the lower abdominals through a count of 10 seconds. Hold and squeeze for 2 seconds at the MTP (when your butt is just off the ground). Lower your body down to starting position through a 10-second count. Without resting, repeat three times.

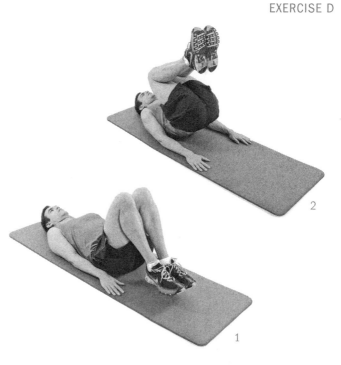

Lateral Squat

Take a stance about a foot wider than shoulder-width on each side. Feather your breathing as you squat down toward one leg, while keeping the opposite leg straight through a count of 10 seconds. Hold for 2 seconds at the MTP. Return to starting position through a count of 10 seconds. Without resting, alternate sides and complete 2 reps on each side for a total of 4.

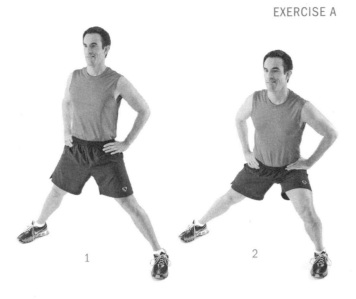

Superman

Lie facedown with your body completely extended, arms parallel to one another, and legs straight. Feather your breathing as you simultaneously lift your arms and your legs through a count of 10 seconds. Hold and squeeze for 2 seconds at the MTP. Return to starting position through a count of 10 seconds. Without resting, repeat three more times. (Note: The range of motion is shorter on this one so be sure to adjust accordingly.)

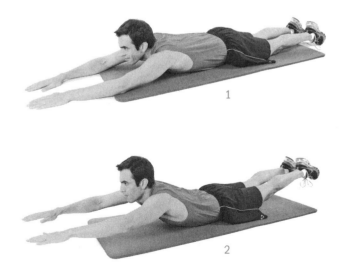

V Push-up

EXERCISE C

Plant feet hip-distance apart. Bend forward at the hips to place hands on the floor 2 to 3 feet in front of your toes. Keep abs drawn in, head tucked like you're holding an orange between your chin and chest (you should look like an upside-down V from the side). With hands slightly in front of your shoulders, feather your breathing as you bend your elbows, lower chest, and shoulders toward the floor through a count of 10 seconds. Hold at the MTP for 2 seconds. Push back to starting position through a count of 10 seconds. Without resting, repeat three more times.

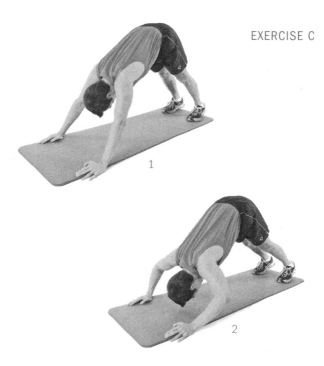

Bicycle Crunch

EXERCISE D

Lie flat on your back. Place your hands behind your head and raise your heels up about 2 inches from the ground, keeping your chin up and abs tight throughout the exercise. Bring your right elbow to your left knee and feather your breathing as you rotate to the other side for a count of 10 seconds. Hold and squeeze for 2 seconds at the MTP (where your left elbow meets your right knee). Lower to starting position through a count of 10 seconds. Without resting, repeat three times.

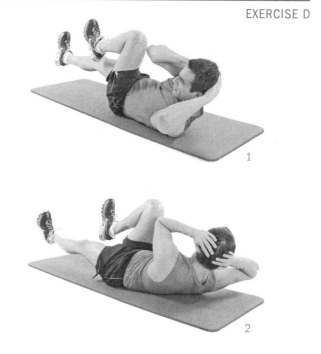

SELECTED BIBLIOGRAPHY

Chapter 1: An Extraordinary Secret

Gosnell, M. "Killer Fat." *Discover,* February 2007.

Ibañez, J., M. Izquierdo, I. Arguelles, et al. "Twice Weekly Progressive Resistance Training Decreases Abdominal Fat and Improves Insulin Sensitivity in Older Men with Type 2 Diabetes." *Diabetes Care* 28 (2005):662–67.

Ormsbee, M. J., J. Thyfault, E. Johnson, et al. "Fat Metabolism and Acute Resistance in Trained Men." *Journal of Applied Physiology* 102 (2007):1767–72.

Richmond, M. "Metabolism: The Calories You Spend." *Northwestern University Fit Bite,* November 2005.

Treuth, M. S., G. R. Hunter, T. Hunter, et al. "Reduction in Intra-Abdominal Adipose Tissue After Strength Training in Older Women." *Journal of Applied Physiology* 78 (1995):1425–31.

Zurlo, F., K. Larson, C. Bogardus, et al. "Skeletal Muscle Metabolism Is a Major Determinant of Resting Energy Expenditure." *Journal of Clinical Investigation* 86 (1990):1423–27.

Chapter 2: The *More* Myth

Burleson, M. A. Jr., H. S. O'Bryant, M. H. Stone, et al., "Effect of Weight Training Exercise and Treadmill Exercise on Postexercise Oxygen Consumption." *Medicine & Science in Sports & Exercise* 30 (1998):518–22.

Chetlin, R. D. "Contemporary Issues in Resistance Training: What Works?" *ACSM Fit Society Page,* Fall 2002:3.

Fry, A. C. "Overtraining with Resistance Exercise." *Current Comment from the ACSM,* January 2001.

Gill, I. P. S., and C. Mbubaegbu. "Fracture Shaft of Clavicle, an Indirect Injury from Bench Pressing." *British Journal of Sports Medicine* 38 (2004):26.

Gillette, C. A., R. C. Bullough, and C. L. Melby. "Postexercise Energy Expenditure in Response to Acute Aerobic or Resistive Exercise." *International Journal of Sport Nutrition and Exercise Metabolism* 4 (1994):347–60.

Goertzen, M., K. Schoppe, G. Lange, et al. "Injuries and Damage Caused by Excess Stress in Body Building and Power Lifting." *Sportverletzung Sportschaden: Organ der Gesellschaft für Orthopädisch-Traumatologische Sportmedizin* 3 (1989):32–36.

Haupt, H. A. "Upper Extremity Injuries Associated with Strength Training." *Clinics in Sports Medicine* 20 (2001):481–90.

Kentta, G., and P. Hassmen. "Overtraining and Recovery. A Conceptual Model." *Sports Medicine* 26 (1998):1–16.

Konig, M., and K. Biener. "Sport-Specific Injuries and Weight Lifting." *Schweizerische Zeitschrift für Sportmedizin* 38 (1990):25–30.

Lombardi, V. P., and R. K. Troxel. "U.S. Deaths & Injuries Associated with Weight Training." *Medicine & Science in Sports & Exercise* 35 (2003):S203.

Mazur, L. J., R. J. Yetman, and W. L. Risser. "Weight-Training Injuries. Common Injuries and Preventative Methods." *Sports Medicine* 16 (1993):57–63.

Montes-Rodriguez, C. J., P. E. Rueda-Orozco, E. Urteaga-Urias, et al. "From Neuronal Recovery to the Reorganisation of Neuronal Circuits: A Review of the Functions of Sleep." *Revista de Neurologia* 43 (2006):409–15.

Osterberg, K. L., and C. L. Melby. "Effect of Acute Resistance Exercise on Postexercise Oxygen Consumption and Resting Metabolic Rate in Young Women." *International Journal of Sport Nutrition and Exercise Metabolism* 10 (2000):360.

Pyron, M. "Overtraining Syndrome." *ACSM Fit Society Page.* Spring 2004:15.

Reynolds, J. M., and L. Kravitz. "Resistance Training and EPOC." *IDEA Personal Trainer* 12 (2001):17–19.

Chapter 3: What Is the 12-Second Sequence™?

Alexander, A., and C. J. De Luca. "Firing Rates of Motor Units in Human Vastus Lateralis Muscle During Fatiguing Isometric Contractions." *Journal of Applied Physiology* 99 (2005):268–80.

Bejeck, B. "All About Abs." *IDEA Health & Fitness Source* 18 (2000):29.

Beltman, J. G. M., A. J. Sargeant, W. van Mechelen, et al. "Voluntary Activation Level and Muscle Fiber Recruitment of Human Quadriceps During Lengthening Contractions." *Journal of Applied Physiology* 97 (2004):619–26.

Chtara, M., K. Chamari, A. Chaouachi, et al. "Effects of Intrasession Concurrent Endurance and Strength Training Sequence on Aerobic Performance and Capacity." *British Journal of Sports Medicine* 39 (2005):555–61.

Cobleigh, B., and I. Kaufer. "Circuit Weight Training—An Answer to Achieving Physical Fitness?" *Journal of Physical Education, Recreation & Dance* 63 (1992):18–24.

Crowther, G. J., and R. K. Gronka. "Fiber Recruitment Affects Oxidative Recovery Measurements of Human Muscle in Vivo." *Medicine & Science in Sports & Exercise* 34 (2002):1733–37.

Cunningham, J. J. "A Reanalysis of the Factors Influencing Basal Metabolic Rate in Normal Adults." *American Journal of Clinical Nutrition* 33 (1980):2372–74.

Darden, E. *The New High Intensity Training.* New York: Rodale, 2004.

Fleck, S. J., and W. J. Kraemer. *Designing Resistance Training Programs.* Champaign, IL: Human Kinetics, 2004.

Fuglevand, A. J., D. A. Winter, and A. E. Patla. "Models of Recruitment and Rate Coding Organization in Motor-Unit Pools." *Journal of Neurophysiology* 70 (1993):2470–88.

Gettman, L. R., and M. L. Pollock. Circuit weight training: A critical review of its physiological benefits. *The Physician and Sportsmedicine* 9 (1981): 44–60.

Goldberg, A. L., J. D. Etlinger, D. F. Goldspink, et al. "Mechanism of Work-Induced Hypertrophy of Skeletal Muscle." *Medicine & Science in Sports & Exercise* 7 (1975):185–98.

Gotshalk, L. A., R. A. Berger, and W. J. Kraemer. "Cardiovascular Responses to a High-Volume Continuous Circuit Resistance Training Protocol." *Journal of Strength and Conditioning Research* 18 (2004):760–64.

Hahn, F., and M. Eades, M.D. *The Slow Burn Fitness Revolution: The Slow-Motion Exercise That Changes Your Body in 30 Minutes a Week.* New York: Random House, 2003.

Haltom, R. W., R. R. Kraemer, R. A. Sloan, et al. "Circuit Weight Training and Its Effects on Excess Postexercise Oxygen Consumption." *Medicine & Science in Sports & Exercise* 31 (1999):1613–18.

Harber, M. P., A. C. Fry, M. R. Rubin, et al. "Skeletal Muscle and Hormonal Adaptations to Circuit Weight Training in Untrained Men." *Scandinavian Journal of Medicine & Science in Sports* 14 (2004):76.

Houtman, C. J., D. F. Stegeman, J. P. Van Dijk, et al. "Changes in Muscle Fiber Conduction Velocity Indicate Recruitment of Distinct Motor Unit Populations." *Journal of Applied Physiology* 95 (2003):1045–54.

Hunter, G. R., D. Seehorst, and S. Snyder. "Comparison of Metabolic and Heart Rate Responses to Super Slow vs. Traditional Resistance Training." *Journal of Strength and Conditioning Research* 17 (2003):76–81.

Jacons, P. L., M. S. Nash, and J. W. Rusinowski. "Circuit Training Provides Cardiorespiratory and Strength Benefits in Persons with Paraplegia." *Medicine & Science in Sports & Exercise* 33 (2001):711–18.

Johnston, B. D. "Moving Too Rapidly in Strength Training Will Unload Muscles and Limit Full Range Strength Development Adaptation: A Case Study." *JEPonline* 8 (2004):36–45.

Kaikkonen, H., M. Yrjämä, E. Siljander, et al. "The Effect of Heart Rate Controlled Low Resistance Circuit Weight Training and Endurance Training on Maximal Aerobic Power in Sedentary Adults." *Scandinavian Journal of Medicine & Science in Sports* 10 (2000):211–15.

Karp, J. R. "Muscle Fiber Types and Training." *Strength and Conditioning Journal* 23 (2001):21–26.

Keeler, L. K., L. H. Finkelstein, W. Miller, et al. "Early Phase Adaptations of Traditional-Speed vs. Super Slow Resistance Training on Strength and Aerobic Capacity in Sedentary Individuals." *Journal of Strength and Conditioning Research* 15 (2001):309–14.

Kravitz, L. "New Insights into Circuit Training." *IDEA Fitness Journal* 4 (2005):24–26.

Little, J. *Advanced Max Contraction Training.* New York: McGraw-Hill, 2006.

———. *Max Contraction Training: The Scientifically Proven Program for Building Muscle Mass in Minimum Time.* New York: McGraw-Hill, 2004.

Little, J., and J. Sharkey. *The Wisdom of Mike Mentzer.* New York: McGraw-Hill, 2005.

McDonagh, M. J., and C. T. Davies. "Adaptive Responses of Mammalian Skeletal Muscle to Exercise with High Loads." *European Journal of Applied Physiology and Occupational Physiology* 52 (1984):139–55.

Mentzer, M., and J. Little. *High-Intensity Training the Mike Mentzer Way.* New York: McGraw-Hill, 2002.

Miller, A. T., and C. S. Blyth. "Lean Body Mass as a Metabolic Reference Standard." *Journal of Applied Physiology* 5 (1953):311–16.

Moen, S. "Circuit Training Through the Muscular System." *Journal of Physical Education, Recreation & Dance* 67 (1996):109–12.

Nelson, J., and L. Kravitz. "Super Slow Resistance Training." *IDEA Personal Trainer* 13 (2002):13–15.

———. "Super Slow Resistance Training: What Does the Research Say?" *IDEA Personal Trainer* 13 (2002): 13–18.

Nelson, M. *Strong Women Stay Slim.* New York: Bantam, 1998.

O'Connor, P., G. Sforzo, and P. Frye. "Effect of Breathing Instruction on Blood Pressure Responses During Isometric Exercise." *Physical Therapy* 69 (1989):757–62.

Philbin, J. *High-Intensity Training.* Champaign, IL: Human Kinetics, 2004.

Poehlman, E. T., M. I. Goran, A. W. Gardner, et al. "Determinants of Decline in Resting Metabolic Rate in Aging Females." *American Journal of Physiology—Endocrinology and Metabolism* 164 (1993): E450–55.

Pratley, R., B. Nicklas, M. Rubin, et al. "Strength Training Increases Resting Metabolic Rate and Norepinephrine Levels in Healthy 50- to 65-Year-Old Men." *Journal of Applied Physiology* 76 (1994):133–37.

Reynolds, J. "Case Study: Weight Loss: A Client Finally Sees Results with a Unique Circuit Training Program." *IDEA Health & Fitness Source* 22 (2004):66–70.

Richmond, M. "Metabolism: The Calories You Spend." *Northwestern University Fit Bite,* November 2005.

Sayers, S. P., J. Bean, A. Cuoco, et al. "Changes in Function and Disability After Resistance Training: Does Velocity Matter?" *American Journal of Physical Medicine & Rehabilitation* 82 (2003):605–13.

Sisco, P., and J. Little. *Static Contraction Training.* New York: Contemporary, 1999.

Smith, L. K., E. L. Weiss, and L. D. Lehmkuhl. *Brunstrom's Clinical Kinesiology.* Philadelphia: F. A. Davis, 1996.

Taafe, D. R., L. Pruitt, G. Pyka, et al. "Comparative Effects of High- and Low-Intensity Resistance Training on Thigh Muscle Strength, Fiber Area, and Tissue Composition in Elderly Women." *Clinical Physiology* 16 (1996):381–92.

Tanimoto, M., and N. Ishii. "Effects of Low-Intensity and Resistance Exercise with Slow Movement and Tonic Force Generation on Muscular Function in Young Men." *Journal of Applied Physiology* 100 (2006):1150–57.

Weider, B. "How Slow Should You Go? What Is Super-Slow Training and Does it Really Work More Muscle Fibers?" *Muscle & Fitness* 65 (2004):194–95.

Weider, J. "Dense, Striated and Cut!" *Muscle & Fitness* 53 (1992):82–88.

Westcott, W. L., R. A. Winett, E. S. Anderson, et al. "Effects of Regular and Slow Speed Resistance Training on Muscle Strength." *Journal of Sports Medicine and Physical Fitness* 41 (2001):154–58.

Williams, P. A., and T. F. Cash. "Effects of a Circuit Weight Training Program on the Body Images of College Students." *International Journal of Eating Disorders* 30 (2001):75–82.

Zickerman, A., and B. Schley. *Power of 10: The Once-a-Week Slow Motion Fitness Revolution.* New York: HarperCollins, 2003.

Zinczenko, D. *The Abs Diet.* New York: Rodale, 2004.

Zurlo, F., K. Larson, C. Bogardus, et al. "Skeletal Muscle Metabolism Is a Major Determinant of Resting Energy Expenditure." *Journal of Clinical Investigation* 86 (1990):1423–27.

Chapter 4: Eating Right

Antoine, J. M., R. Rohr, M. J. Gagery, R. E. Bleyer, and G. Debry. "Feeding Frequency and Nitrogen Balance in Weight-reduction Obese Women." *Human Nutrition: Clinical Nutrition* 38, no. 1 (1984):313–38.

Boirie, Y., M. Dangin, P. Gachon, et al. "Slow and Fast Dietary Proteins Differently Modulate Postprandial Protein Accretion." *Proceedings of the National Academy of Sciences of the United States of America* 94 (1997):14930–35.

Bushman, J. L. "Green Tea and Cancer in Humans: A Review of the Literature." *Nutrition and Cancer* 31 (1998):151–59.

Craig, W. J. "Health-Promoting Properties of Common Herbs." *American Journal of Clinical Nutrition* 70 (1999):419S–499S.

Dangin, M., Y. Boirie, C. Guillet, et al. "Influence of the Protein Digestion Rate on Protein Turnover in Young and Elderly Subjects." *Journal of Nutrition* 132 (2002):3228S–3233S.

Dauncey, M. J., and S. A. Bingham. "Dependence of 24 h Energy Expenditure in Man on the Composition of the Nutrient Intake." *British Journal of Nutrition* 50 (1983):1–13.

Farshchi, H. R., M. A. Taylor, and I. A. Macdonald. "Decreased Thermic Effect of Food after an Irregular Compared with a Regular Meal Pattern in Healthy Lean Women." *International Journal of Obesity Related Metabolic Disorders* 28, no. 5 (2004): 653–60.

Fogteloo, A. J., H. Pijl, F. Roelfsema, M. Frölich, and A. E. Meinders. "Impact of Meal Timing and Frequency on the Twenty-four-hour Leptin Rhythm." *Hormone Research* 62, no. 2 (2004):71–78.

Garrow, J. S. "The Contribution of Protein Synthesis to Thermogenesis in Man." *International Journal of Obesity* 9 (1985):97–101.

Graham, H. N. "Green Tea Composition, Consumption, and Polyphenol Chemistry." *Preventive Medicine* 21 (1992):334–50.

Hall, W. L., Millward D. J., Long, S. J., et al. "Casein and Whey Exert Different Effects on Plasma Amino Acid Profiles, Gastrointestinal Hormone Secretion and Appetite." British Journal of Nutrition 89 (2003):239–48.

Hutchins, K. SuperSlow®: The ULTIMATE Exercise Protocol. Castleberry, FL: Media Support by Ken Hutchins, 1989.

Imai, K., K. Suga, and K. Nakachi. "Cancer Preventive Effects of Drinking Green Tea Among a Japanese Population." *Preventive Medicine* 26 (1997):769–75.

Iwao, S., K. Mori, and Y. Sato. "Effects of Meal Frequency on Body Composition During Weight Control in Boxers." *Scandinavian Journal of Medicine & Science in Sports* 6, no. 5 (1996):265–72.

Katiyar, S., C. A. Elmets, and S. K. Katiyar. "Green Tea and Skin Cancer: Photoimmunology, Angiogenesis, and DNA Repair." *Journal of Nutritional Biochemistry* (2006):Epub (ahead of print).

Mikkelson, P. B., S. Toubro, and A. Astrup. "Effect of Fat-Reduced Diets on 24-h Energy Expenditure: Comparisons Between Animal Protein, Vegetable Protein, and Carbohydrate." *American Journal of Clinical Nutrition* 72 (2000):1135–41.

Millward, D. J., P. J. Garlick, R. J. Stewart, et al. "Skeletal-Muscle Growth and Protein Turnover." *Biochemical Journal* 150 (1975):235–43.

Mirkov, S., B. J. Komoroski, J. Ramirez, et al. "Effects of Green Tea Compounds on Irinotecan Metabolism." *Drug Metabolism and Disposition* (2006):Epub (ahead of print).

Murphy, M. "Feed the Fat Furnace: Chicken, Fish, and Protein Powders Can Help You Build Muscle and Burn Away Fat." *Men's Fitness,* October 2003.

Nagle, D. G., D. Ferreira, and Y. D. Zhou. "Epigallocatechin-3-Gallate (EGCG): Chemical and Biomedical Perspectives." *Phytochemistry* 67 (2006)1849–55.

Nestel, P. J., S. E. Pomeroy, T. Sasahara, et al. "Arterial Compliance in Obese Subjects Is Improved with Dietary Plant n-3 Fatty Acid from Flaxseed Oil Despite Increased LDL Oxidizability." *Arteriosclerosis, Thrombosis, and Vascular Biology* 17 (1999):1163–70.

PDRhealth. Drug Information: L-glutamine. http://www.pdrhealth.com/drug_info/nmdrugprofiles/nutsupdrugs/lgl_0125.shtml

Raben, A., L. Agerhold-Larson, A. Flint, et al. "Meals with Similar Energy Densities But Rich in Protein, Fat, Carbohydrate, or Alcohol Have Different Effects on Energy Expenditure and Substrate Metabolism But Not on Appetite and Energy Intake." *American Journal of Clinical Nutrition* 77 (2003):91–100.

Robinson, S. M., C. Jaccard, C. Persaud, et al. "Protein Turnover and Thermogenesis in Response to High-Protein and High-Carbohydrate Feeding in Men." *American Journal of Clinical Nutrition* 52 (1990):72–80.

Segal, K. R., B. Gutin, A. M. Nyman, et al. "Thermic Effect of Food at Rest, During Exercise, and After Exercise in Lean and Obese Men of Similar Body Weight." *Journal of Clinical Investigation* 76 (1985):1107–12.

Tipton, K. D., B. B. Rasmussen, S. L. Miller, et al. "Timing of Amino Acid–Carbohydrate Ingestion Alters Anabolic Response of Muscle to Resistance to Exercise." *American Journal of Physiology* 281 (2001):E197–E206.

Tipton, K. D., and R. R. Wolfe. "Exercise, Protein Metabolism, and Muscle Growth." *International Journal of Sport Nutrition and Exercise Metabolism* 11 (2001):109–32.

Westerterp-Plantenga, M. S., M. P. G. M. Lejune, I. Nijs, et al. "High Protein Intake Sustains Weight Maintenance After Body Weight Loss in Humans." *International Journal of Obesity* 28 (2004):57–64.

Ziegler, T. R., K. Benfell, R. J. Smith, et al. "Safety and Metabolic Effects of L-Glutamine Administration in Humans." *Journal of Parenteral and Enteral Nutrition* 14 (1990):137S–146S.

ABOUT THE AUTHOR

Jorge Cruise personally struggled with weight as a child and a young man. Today he is recognized as America's leading wellness expert for busy people. He is the author of two *New York Times* bestsellers: *8 Minutes in the Morning®,* published in fourteen languages, and *The 3-Hour Diet™*. Jorge coaches clients daily at 12second.com and 3hourdiet.com. He can be found offering advice and coaching online at AOL.com and lifescript.com. Each Sunday, his *USA WEEKEND* magazine column reaches more than 51 million readers in six hundred newspapers nationwide. He has appeared on *Oprah,* CNN, *Good Morning America, Today, Extra, The Tyra Banks Show, Dateline NBC,* VH1, and *The View.* You can contact Jorge at jorgecruise.com.

12-SECOND SEQUENCE™
APPROVED PRODUCTS

I have tested a lot of products, and the following are my favorites. In fact, they're the only products to carry my exclusive 12-Second Sequence™ seal. For more information on these products, visit 12second.com.

BALLY® TOTAL FITNESS

I love Bally® because they've got a lot of experience in the fitness industry (more than forty years) and they are in over 350 convenient locations across the country. Whether I'm at my home in California or traveling to the East Coast, Bally® Total Fitness is always easy to get to. And the great thing about Bally's® is that you can get a free 12-Second Sequence™ class when you download the pass from 12second.com. Plus, there are more than five thousand trainers at Bally® locations across the country who have been trained in the 12-Second Sequence™ method, so you're guaranteed great form and technique.

BARLEAN'S® FLAXSEED OIL

All Barlean's® products are completely fresh and organic. Freshness is absolutely key, because flaxseed oil goes rancid very quickly—and when it's rancid, it tastes awful! I love it and take it every day, and one of my son Parker's favorite snacks is Barlean's® Flaxseed Oil on toast.

- Original
- Lignan
- Flavored (Cinnamon, Lemonade)
- Forti-Flax
- Greens

GOFIT™

I love GoFit™'s products because they are convenient, safe, and comfortable. For example, their Sportblock® combines 8 pairs of dumbbells into one space-saving, easy-to-hold design. Their exercise ball is burst-resistant up to 500 pounds, which means that you'll never have to worry about your safety while exercising with it. Finally, their Pilates® mat is the softest, most comfortable mat out there. These three products are the ones that are featured in the exercises in this book.

- Sportblock® Adjustable Dumbbell Set and Sportblock Add-on Weight Set
- Pilates® mat
- Exercise Balls (55 cm, 65 cm, and 75 cm)
- Abwheel

- Power Tubes
- Power Flat Bands
- Weighted Toning Balls
- Multi-Tube Gym

JORGE'S PACKS™ VITAMINS

One of my favorite things about these vitamins is that they come in single-serving, personalized packets—they even have your name printed on each little pack. They're portable and great for travel and everyday use. Plus, they contain everything that's right for you based on your custom online profile. I take mine with me everywhere I go!

JORGE'S PACKS™ WHEY PROTEIN POWDER

Jorge's Packs™ protein shakes are my favorite because they taste great and are rich in nutrients. They are delicious and the only ones that I drink each day as my three snacks. I love all the flavors (chocolate, strawberry, vanilla), but my favorite is chocolate. It tastes just like chocolate milk. Available exclusively online at jorgespacks.com.

PRECOR®

Precor's machines are absolutely top-quality. When you're investing in a home gym, you want to make sure that your equipment is durable, reliable, and engineered to move the way you move. Precor's products are carefully designed with human movement in mind, which make them the smoothest, most ergonomic machines you can buy. The S3.23 Functional Trainer Cable Machine is the one featured in this book and the one I use personally at home.

- S3.23 Functional Trainer Cable Machine

- 9.35 Treadmill

INDEX

12-Second Sequence™
WORKOUT DVD

Get your best body ever!

Burn Fat…
Build Muscle…
**See Results in Two
Weeks!**

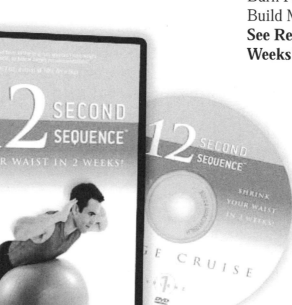

Available Now!

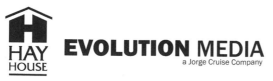

12-Second Sequence™ Journal

This journal provides inspirational quotes and daily meditations to help keep you motivated throughout your 8-Week Challenge. You'll also find daily eating and workout logs to keep you on track, as well as helpful nutritional tips and on-the-go eating guides. Available everywhere books are sold.

12-Second Sequence™ Audiobook

Jorge takes you through the science and theory behind the 12-Second Sequence™ in this audio recording that makes it easy for you to understand the principles outlined in the core book. This audiobook is the perfect solution for beginners or people who just don't have the time to read the core book. Available everywhere books are sold.

12-Second Sequence™ [Spanish edition]

Do you know a Spanish-speaker who needs to get in shape? *La Secuencia de 12 Segundos*™ is the perfect gift for a friend who wants to get fit, eat smart, and achieve his or her ideal body. Available everywhere books are sold.